FEED THEM WELL

FEED THEM WELL

A Guide to Raising Healthy, Confident Eaters for Life

JENNIFER ANDERSON, MSPH, RDN

FLATIRON BOOKS
NEW YORK

This book is intended as a source of information and should not be used as a substitute for professional medical advice or other healthcare. If you have any concerns or questions about any aspect of your child's health, or are considering a new healthcare or nutritional regimen, you should seek the advice of a professional healthcare provider.

The case studies discussed in this book are illustrative and reflect composites based on the author's years of experience rather than the experiences of any particular person. Elsewhere in the text, some names and identifying details have been changed.

Printed in the United States of America. For information, address Flatiron Books, 120 Broadway, New York, NY 10271. EU Representative: Macmillan Publishers Ireland Ltd., 1st Floor, The Liffey Trust Centre, 117–126 Sheriff Street Upper, Dublin 1, D01 YC43.

www.flatironbooks.com

The Library of Congress Cataloging-in-Publication Data is available upon request.

ISBN 978-1-250-38773-8 (hardcover)
ISBN 978-1-250-38774-5 (ebook)

First Edition: 2026

10 9 8 7 6 5 4 3 2 1

To my mom, Lora, who transforms people with love, health, connection, and hope—by feeding them

CONTENTS

FEED THEM WELL

INTRODUCTION

Before I had kids, I was confident that when I *did* become a parent, feeding my child would be simple. After all, I'm a registered dietitian. I have a master's degree in public health. I've worked as a nutrition consultant to the US Department of Agriculture, reviewing education initiatives from all over the country. Surely, it wouldn't be that hard to feed my own child!

So when my son was born, the plan was straightforward: no added sugars or processed foods for two years. I would make all of his food, and he would, of course, love it. I was wholly confident in this plan until my son was three months into eating solid foods. At a well visit weigh-in, our pediatrician uttered the sentence every new parent dreads: "He's not gaining weight."

I felt like a failure. My son was born a chunky baby, his cheeks plump and kissable. But then he learned to crawl and started walking, and he didn't want to sit and eat. He wanted to play! This seemed like age-appropriate, growing-kid behavior, so I didn't think all that much of it until that day in the pediatrician's office. Suddenly, my son's eating became *all* I thought about. Most parents (especially moms, I find) go into this job believing that at a bare minimum, we should be good at feeding our children. We've been doing it since the dawn of time! It feels like our most basic, most primal, responsibility. Now, every day, I was plagued with questions: *Did he eat enough? Is he getting what he needs? Am I failing him?*

I armed myself with as much information as I could, diving

into the best practices for feeding kids, consulting our pediatrician, other parents, and a plethora of research articles and books. My husband and I committed to applying what I'd learned, and we devised many of our own hacks. I remember making a list of high-calorie foods and posting it on the refrigerator. The rule was: We had to add something high calorie to every meal or snack we served our son. It was a lot of work. And a lot of worry. Nothing keeps a parent up at night like anxiety over their child's well-being.

Eventually, my son got back on track with his expected weight gain. But a few years later, he started preschool, which meant he'd be eating one meal and two snacks in a more distracting environment. My anxiety surrounding his diet returned, and so I took on a new task: finding food options that he would be willing to eat on his own in the busy preschool classroom. I started making little bento box lunches for him to take to school. These were colorful, high-calorie meals that included star-shaped cheese cutouts, applesauce mixed with ground nuts, and cute little food picks added. I put *a lot* of effort into creating those bento boxes. I figured that if I could capture my son's attention and make his lunches fun and visually appealing, I could probably get him to eat them.

One day, a friend who saw my lunches suggested I start an Instagram page. I thought that if the hacks I'd created and the information I'd amassed could help other parents, it was well worth the effort of posting some photos of them on social media. Alongside each lunch photo I posted, I included my tips for feeding kids and helping them learn to eat more foods. Almost immediately, the account caught parents' attention. People started sharing it, my audience grew, and I quickly learned that many other parents out there were having a similarly tough time feeding their kids. Before I knew it, Kids Eat in Color had become a thriving and encouraging place for parents to get evidence-based resources on feeding their kids.

In the early days of KEIC, picky eating was the most common

concern shared by parents. They wondered about their baby's refusal of food, their toddler suddenly eating a fraction of what they ate before, their preschooler refusing foods they had always liked, or their school-age kid coming home with a full lunchbox they had hardly touched.* However, as the KEIC community has grown, and the food environment surrounding us has become increasingly complex, noisy, and confusing, many parents are looking for additional guidance that goes well beyond strategies for how to handle picky eating. They want to know what their kids should eat to prevent or reverse disease. They worry about whether processed foods and additives are poisoning their children. More parents have children with health conditions, and they wonder what changes they need to make to their child's diet. What kids are (or aren't) eating is at the forefront of parents' minds.

Amid all the concern about nutrition, many parents are also deeply concerned about their child's relationship with food and their body. They don't want their child to base their self-worth on their body size and take on the burden of endless weight-loss diets and disordered eating. I once received a DM from a woman who was worried about her three-year-old niece. The girl's grandfather had offered her a piece of chocolate, and the response from the little girl was startling. "I can't eat it," she said. "I'll get fat." Parents share stories like this and worry that their child won't have a peaceful relationship with their body or be able to enjoy food.

So yes, as parents, we have a lot of fears surrounding how we feed our kids. Let's take a closer look at how we got here, why the simple task of feeding our kids has become such a challenge, and how the stakes have grown so high.

---

* When I say *picky eating*, I'm not talking about a character trait. I've seen parents get annoyed at their kid and say, "Ugh, he's being so picky!" When I use the phrase *picky eating*, I'm referring to a behavior—a kid rejecting a lot of foods for any reason.

THE TROUBLE WITH OUR FOOD ENVIRONMENT

In the US, and around the world, food and beverage corporations that prioritize profits over the health of consumers have gained an outsize influence on the way we eat in the absence of governmental regulation. This is especially true when it comes to our children. In the US alone, these companies spend *billions of dollars* annually on food marketing to kids and about $14 billion a year on food marketing total, which also affects kids. Their goal is simple: to get children hooked on their products. And it works. The more kids are exposed to food marketing, the more likely they are to eat the foods marketed.

As just one example, the other day, I walked down the granola bar aisle at Target with my head at my child's eye level. What did I see? Box after box of packaged snacks emblazoned with cartoon characters, bright colors, and images of smiling, happy kids. Food marketing to children has become so ubiquitous that often we don't even notice it—we see it on TV and online, on toys and clothing. We see it via schools in the à la carte snack options and food packaging for items served as part of national school meal programs and nutrition education curricula. Adults who grew up in the '80s and '90s probably remember cereal box characters like Snap, Crackle, and Pop, or Tony the Tiger, with fondness. Today, this type of food marketing seems almost quaint, as companies have continued to use food engineering to make their products more "addictive" and improved food marketing to be more psychologically manipulative. Food companies run thousands of tests to find the exact amount of sugar, salt, fat, and sensory properties that a product must contain to encourage people to eat more of it. Companies then use this data to create bright, fun "hyperpalatable foods," defined as highly processed foods that are designed to be difficult to stop eating. "Once you pop, you can't stop," one brand of chips promises. If you've ever experienced a *perfectly* chewy gummy bear, *perfectly* bubbly soda, or *perfectly* crunchy chip, you've experienced hyperpalatability. These hyperpalatable foods may be laden with dyes and additives, or they may be organic and additive-free. Regardless, they are addictively tasty and very easy to like on the first bite.

Before I go further, I want to emphasize that while these hyperpalatable foods make our food environment tricky to navigate, I don't believe that foods are categorically "good" or "bad." This is a message that we will return to—that foods are not "good" or "bad"; they do different things in our bodies. This is incredibly important to keep in mind when talking to your kids about food. Foods are different from each other, but we don't need to constantly live in fear about what our kids are eating. And yet—we can't understand what we're up against as parents, without understanding the influence of our food environment and acknowledging certain realities.

In the United States, hyperpalatable foods make up over 56 percent of young children's diets, and over 60 percent of the diets of six-to-eighteen-year-olds. These foods tend to be low in protein, dietary fiber, micronutrients (vitamins and minerals), and phytochemicals (plant compounds that do helpful things in our bodies). Beyond lacking nutrients, these foods may contain contaminants or additives from processing and packaging. And hyperpalatable foods tend to alter eating patterns, promote snacking, change the speed of eating, and result in absent-minded and compulsive eating. These factors also influence digestion and the brain processes involved in feeling satisfied after a meal or snack and are associated with pediatric health conditions.

We want our children to listen to their bodies, eat when they are hungry, and stop when they are full. But the pleasure of eating hyperpalatable foods activates the reward system in a person's brain, which often leads to eating more of the hyperpalatable food than we would have compared with a "boring" food. Think about a vegetable you like and how you feel when you first bite into it. Now, think about your favorite dessert or snack and how you feel with that first bite. I love a good, crisp carrot, but it doesn't hit the same as a salty, kettle-cooked potato chip. Not only are hyperpalatable foods more rewarding than "boring" foods, they also change children's brains, in some cases permanently determining a child's food preferences or their future risk for overeating. This is especially relevant during periods of rapid development. And while different children will be affected to different degrees, all children are susceptible.

Food marketing isn't the only factor making our food environment challenging for parents. "Diet culture" and the idea that *thinner is better* is represented everywhere we look, from social media to TV to video games to music and movies. When kids internalize the idea that thin is ideal, they develop *weight bias*, which can lead to rejecting, stigmatizing, or assigning less value to people they perceive to have a higher weight. Some children show bias against people of higher weights as young as two, three, and four years old. They often turn this weight stigma on themselves, in what's referred to as *internalized weight bias*. Children with more internalized weight bias are more likely to be unhappy with their own bodies and struggle with depression, anxiety, and other physical and emotional problems. They are more likely to develop restrictive eating, eating disorders, guilt and preoccupation with food, and to put themselves on a weight-loss diet.

Weight stigma doesn't only come from media sources—it also comes from friends, family, and healthcare providers. The weight-management industry, which is projected to be worth more than $295 billion by 2027, depends on it. Even the medical and pharmaceutical industries benefit from it, pushing the thin ideal for economic gain. With the rise in availability of GLP-1 inhibitors (medications used for weight loss) for adults and children, the thin ideal has become even more lucrative for these industries. Parents are up against all of this mess that diet culture creates, and it's not a fair fight.

The truth is, we are facing a national childhood health crisis, one that imperils our kids' mental and physical health. In the past three decades, we've seen an uptick in the number of children with diseases related to diet and nutrition—like type 2 diabetes, hypertension, and eating disorders. When we view this health crisis through a wider lens, we see the forces of diet culture, food marketing, and a profit-driven food system at work. These forces are bigger than any individual family. We cannot and should not have to fight them alone. They will require governmental regulation to see lasting improvement. Although we might hear promises from private industry to improve the food system, their track record on such promises, including one to reduce food marketing to children, assures us they are empty promises. I believe we should advocate for policy changes. We need regulations to limit children's exposure to food and wellness marketing (including the marketing of GLP-1 inhibitors for weight loss), agricultural policies that support fruit and vegetable growth, school food nutrition policies, and environmental policies that keep heavy metals and chemicals out of our food, water, and soil. However, policy change can take decades of advocacy.

In the meantime, since it's up to us, we need a doable approach to teaching our kids to eat in a way that supports their health and preserves a positive relationship with food and their bodies. This includes what we can do as parents to teach and model how to make choices that nourish us, feel good about our bodies, and develop a healthy relationship with food. And while it may seem daunting given all the noise around us, we have what it takes to raise kids who have the knowledge and courage they need to feed themselves meaningfully for a lifetime.

IT'S NOT ABOUT PERFECTION

Our goal is to feed our kids well. But what does that mean? It's not about getting it all right. Our food environment is so mentally and physically toxic that any choice we make can feel risky—and holding ourselves to an imaginary standard of perfection is downright impossible. When I talk about feeding our children *well*, I'm talking about doing our best, making this journey a family affair that we can actively engage in with our kids, and having the courage to make changes when things aren't going as we'd hoped. It can be scary to trust yourself to explore what's best for your family. It can also be scary to make choices that go against the grain of what you've heard that you "should" be doing. However, it's important, above all, to make choices that meet the needs of your individual family. For one family, that might mean eating certain nutrients or following a specific food plan. For another family, it could mean cooking meals from scratch and avoiding all hyperpalatable foods. And for yet another family, it could mean buying more prepared convenience foods and having a liberal hyperpalatable food policy. "Well" is subjective—it is an ever-changing goal you define based on the kids you have, the life you have, and the resources you have.

An integral piece of feeding our children well is teaching them to eat with "embodied independence," which I'll discuss in more detail in chapter 2. But I want to highlight this concept from the start, because it is so important. When they eat with embodied independence, it means that they are able to trust and be connected to their physical bodies (the embodiment piece), while at the same time keeping in mind the life skills and nutrition information they'll need to take care of those bodies for a lifetime (the independence piece). We won't be cutting their grapes or packing their nut-free sandwiches forever. As parents, we want to nurture embodied independence in our kids so that they can think practically about nutrition as they live in their bodies and go off into the world to navigate an endless decision tree of food choices. Kids who have developed a sense of embodied independence will know that they need a variety of foods in their diet, but they won't tie their internal *value* as a human being to what they eat. Embodied eaters can find joy in food and peace in their bodies, while keeping the basics of health and nutrition in mind.

I find that parents too often think about their kids' diets in extreme terms. Many of the parents in my community feel that if they're not doing the very best for their kids, all the time, then they're doing the worst. But that's not backed by research, and that's not how feeding works. There are general best practices, but every kid—and every family—is different. It's okay to make mistakes and then to look back on these mistakes and realize that a different strategy probably would have been a better fit. That's how we learn.

Your child has a unique body with unique needs, and as they grow, they are going to be shaped by factors outside of your control. They will run into food-related challenges if they haven't already—that's just part of modern life. You may have a kindergartener who ate every veggie on their plate until school lunches entered the picture, or a newly minted adolescent who ate with pleasure and abandon until their peers began talking about portion size. You already know that the only constant in parenting is change. Here's the other thing I want you to know: You have what it takes to support your child through these changes. After all, you're here, reading. You care. You look for solutions when you need them. You are learning to be the parent that your child needs.

HOW TO USE THIS BOOK

You could spend endless hours online brushing up on the best way to solve your latest food drama, but that wouldn't change the fact that following all that expert guidance in real life with real children is complicated. This book is designed to simplify the task of feeding your family—by quieting the noise, streamlining the complex, and when all else fails, showing you how to pivot. In the pages that follow, I will share two evidence-based frameworks I have developed—based on my training in public health, nutrition, and anthropology; my experience educating millions of parents; and my own lived experience as a parent—to help guide you through your food-related decision-making and challenges.

In part 1, "The Five Pillars of Eating with Embodied Independence," I will offer practices for teaching your kids to become independent, embodied eaters (even when you're not there) and helping them to establish a balanced, healthy, and positive relationship with food. But remember, there is no "best way" of feeding children. What works for one family won't necessarily work for another, and the five pillars are meant to be used as fundamentals that you can adapt and personalize to make the best choices for *your* kid and *your* family. These pillars include approaching mealtime with a sense of curiosity; eating together and connecting through food; talking positively about food and bodies; and knowing what to prioritize when it comes to nutrition. I want you to think of each of the five pillars as a practice that you and your child will actively engage in together. Together, the pillars become an entirely new framework for engaging in the "how we feed our kids" discussion, one that is *not* rooted in "you *must* do this" or "you *cannot* do that."

In part 2, "A Six-Step Plan for Navigating Food Dilemmas," I want to empower you with a decision-making system that you can use in especially difficult circumstances. Food dilemmas are situations that force parents to make hard choices. Maybe you feel forced to choose between protecting your child's relationship with food and enforcing specific dietary restrictions to manage their health condition. Maybe you have a child who struggles with gauging their fullness and is so picky they eat only ten foods, which leaves you wondering whether teaching them to trust their body's signals is the best choice. When faced with a food dilemma, you will have to *not* do something that you were told you *should* do. Often, parents facing food dilemmas find themselves unable to follow the "best practices," and they're left feeling overwhelmed, discouraged, and misunderstood. I've been in this position myself; I get it, and I want to give you more options. You will need more creative feeding solutions than the average parent, and part 2 will help you find them.

If the five pillars introduced in part 1 are about building a foundation over time that will allow your child to eat well as they grow, the plan in part 2 is about problem-solving and addressing feeding challenges in real time as they arise. Many of us are dealing with ongoing, unsolvable dinner table dilemmas like severe allergies and disordered eating. The framework in part 2 gives parents the tools to problem-solve based on their family's unique needs, which often involves redefining what "well" looks like for your child. Part 2 will give you a new way of thinking about maneuvering through sticky food dilemmas. In this section, we will also tackle common situations that parents find particularly challenging, including picky eating (both extreme and typical), handling dessert and "junk food," helping a child who is being influenced by diet culture, addressing grandparents or other relatives who don't agree with your approach, and more.

This isn't a book that is full of all the easy or "right" answers. Nothing about this is easy! My family struggles, too. We don't follow every practice in this book every single day—far from it. But we keep them all in mind, and we do our best with the energy and resources and circumstances we're dealing with at any particular moment. It's possible that what worked for your family one day may not work the next, and some strategies will need to be modified over time. Still, this book will give you the tools to navigate complicated moments as your child matures. *Feed Them Well* is about raising a generation of kids who won't internalize all the food noise and anxiety that we, their parents, grew up with. Instead, we want our children to be able to trust their bodies and the lifestyle practices we have instilled in them, giving them a resilient experience of health that will serve them for a lifetime.

After reading this book, you will know how to courageously support your child in their eating journey. You will make decisions based not on fearmongering headlines or popular expert recommendations but on who *you* are and who *they* are. And when it comes to parenting, that's the best practice of all.

PART I

THE FIVE PILLARS OF EATING WITH EMBODIED INDEPENDENCE

1

FEED WITH CURIOSITY

This is a practical, how-to book that is full of recommendations and advice on how to feed your child. However, as we've touched on, there are many ways to approach this task. The recommendations in this book are based on the latest research and data, my personal experience as a parent, and what I've observed educating families, but no one can know better than you do what will work best for *your* family. When it comes to feeding kids, change is a constant. Kids are always growing and changing, and the best practices based on research also change. With all of this in mind, how do we actually determine whether what we are doing is best for our kids? We do this by embracing curiosity—both in the way we think about feeding our kids and the strategies we try out. This is the first pillar of our framework.

At the end of the day, we want to raise kids who are confident and resilient. We want our kids to be able to make decisions for themselves, manage their emotions, and be both physically and mentally healthy. We want them to love themselves. Leading with curiosity means that you are making decisions with these goals in mind. You are thinking about *who your child is* and who you are, and how the feeding decisions you make today can help them grow into the confident, resilient, healthy individuals that you know they can be. When you practice feeding with curiosity, you are asking questions like, "What am I seeing in my child when I only offer meals and snacks at certain times? Does my child's behavior/attitude toward food change? Is that change helpful or unhelpful? Have my thoughts or behaviors changed as I enforce this new structure? Is that change helpful or unhelpful?" By embracing curiosity, we allow ourselves to become more flexible regarding nutrition and meals without constantly second-guessing ourselves.

Before we can begin to practice curiosity, we need to bring a curious perspective to feeding practices in general. Today, we have instantaneous access to an overwhelming amount of research and information via the internet, social media platforms, and AI. And yet, with all this information at our fingertips, we find ourselves increasingly confused, particularly when the advice we hear from influential people is conflicting. How can it be that our trusted sources disagree on what's "right" while also claiming that their advice is backed by *the research*? The answer to this lies in understanding the research process and what research can and cannot tell us.

With the proliferation of food recommendations, feeding trends, and experts warning of the health risks of different foods, it's easy to get stuck in a place of guilt, fear, or even just blindly following the latest trends. However, if you learn how to read the health headlines with an understanding of how research works more generally, and a curiosity about how it will affect your family more specifically, it will serve you in a big way. And it might be easier than it seems.

UNDERSTANDING "THE RESEARCH"

As a parent, you've undoubtedly encountered food-related headlines that begin with phrases like "New research finds . . ." or "Reports say . . ." followed by advice on the next superfood to incorporate in your child's diet or the next toxic additive to avoid. Some of the people writing these headlines have good intentions. Others are simply using the "research" to manipulate you into giving them your money, attention, likes, or political will. We assume that when a health claim is supported by "research," this means that a scientist has tested a bunch of strategies and is reporting on the results of what works with absolute certainty. We assume that researchers can tell us, definitively, what is true for all people and that by following their advice, we'll be doing what's best for our kids. There's a big problem with this assumption, though: It's just not how scientific research works. Research is like a bucket. Individual research studies are drops in that bucket. As the bucket fills, a consensus on a particular health topic may emerge that either informs the general recommendations on this topic or inspires further investigation on this topic. Protein research is a good example. At one point in time, researchers wanted to know how many grams of protein children needed to eat, so they researched it. The drops went into the bucket and a consensus of the protein requirement calculations emerged, and also, after some time passed, some researchers had more questions and saw the opportunity for more investigation. They conducted new research, using different, more modern methods. A few drops from this newer research also went into the bucket. It did not support the consensus protein needs calculations and was also not enough to fully change the consensus. It can be very dangerous to change consensus, beliefs, or actions based on one or two studies. "New study" doesn't always mean "better study." When we look closely at individual research studies, they aren't perfect and they don't all agree, which is the reality of science. And this is okay, because we look at what's in the bucket. That's how science is supposed to work. The new researchers who study protein have said more research is needed, and those keeping up with this topic, like me, know that more information is to come on the topic of protein needs (and you'll see ranges of protein needs discussed in this book to capture the nuance about protein research). Now, when someone tells you about a "research study," you can pause and think, *They are telling me about one drop in the bucket; it's not going to mean much unless they tell me what else is in the bucket.*

OBSERVATIONAL STUDIES: DO PRESCHOOLERS WHO READ FUN BOOKS ABOUT VEGGIES EAT MORE VEGGIES?

Eating with curiosity means we know enough about research to have a healthy respect for its benefits, understand its limitations, and get better at spotting when people are using it irresponsibly. Child feeding research has a lot of limitations, more than in many other fields, such as medicine. It is still valuable, however, if we are willing to embrace a basic understanding of what it can and cannot tell us. This begins with knowing the difference between the two main types of research studies (there are lots of subtypes, but I'll spare you the details on those).

The first type of research study is *observational*. Observational studies simply look at what is without intervening in any way, and they cannot determine if one factor causes an outcome. The vast majority of child feeding research is observational and only describes relationships between things (this is called *correlation*).

Consider this imagined scenario: A group of researchers wonder if kids who read fun books about fruits and veggies eat more veggies. Could this be an easy way to get kids eating more veggies? The researchers design an observational study to start exploring this topic.

In this scenario, let's say the researchers send out surveys to one hundred parents. They ask the parents if they read fun books about fruits and veggies to their preschooler and how many veggies their preschooler eats. The researchers learn that of the kids whose parents read them fun books about fruits and veggies, most of them eat more veggies than the national average, some of them eat the same amount as the national average, and a few of them eat fewer than the national average. The researchers summarize their findings by saying, "Kids whose caregivers read them fun books about fruits and veggies are more likely to eat more of these foods than the national average." Researchers don't know why they have observed this correlation. Maybe kids who love to eat veggies want to be read books about veggies. Who knows! But that's okay, because that's the nature of observational studies. The researchers then publish their findings in a peer-reviewed* journal, which makes it part of the research bucket.

EXPERIMENTAL STUDIES: CAN READING YOUR CHILD A BOOK MAKE THEM EAT MORE VEGGIES?

We'll continue with our research scenario. Another group of researchers is intrigued by the research about books and veggie eating. They want to use the second major type of study, an *experimental* study, to determine whether one thing *causes* something else. For example, these researchers might wonder, "If we read preschoolers a storybook in which a bunny eats carrots and then give the kids carrots for a snack, will they eat more carrots?" So they plan and conduct an experiment to find out. In this experimental study, a researcher reads one hundred preschoolers the story about the bunny who ate carrots, then they serve them a snack of carrots. They also serve a different group of other preschoolers a snack of carrots, but with no story first.

Rather than getting a very simple answer "yes, the kids all ate more carrots" (which is what we parents want), they get *research results*, which look like the following: The researchers find that seventy kids ate *more* carrots after they heard the story, thirty kids ate *fewer* carrots, and ten kids had no change at all. The research team concludes that reading preschoolers a story about carrot-eating bunnies can cause some of them to eat more carrots.

---

* *Peer-reviewed* means that other researchers read and analyzed this paper before it was accepted into a journal and published. Reviewers send changes back to the authors about what they did wrong that they need to fix before it can be published. While not a perfect process, it helps reduce the release of poor information.

They publish their study, and it becomes a drop in the bucket of other studies about books and preschooler veggie eating.

HOW RESEARCH TURNS INTO (IMPERFECT) RECOMMENDATIONS

In this veggie-book scenario, there might be multiple research groups studying whether books play a role in kids' eating. And the studies won't all get the same results. When we look in that research bucket, we will see studies that make different observations and experimental studies that see different results. It's normal for the results of studies in any social science field to disagree. Over time, however, as more observational and especially experimental studies are conducted, it may become apparent that most researchers conclude kids are more likely to eat veggies after they read fun books that feature them. As a result, professionals like registered dietitians or nurses see a consensus and may begin to feel confident telling parents that they should read their child books with fruits and veggies in them. They make this recommendation in the hopes that more kids *in total* will eat more veggies, even though they know many children won't be affected, and some may even eat fewer veggies. These experiments haven't uncovered *why* some kids eat more veggies after veggie stories, but given the information they do have, it would be irresponsible to tell parents to stop reading fun books about fruits and veggies to their kids. So professionals recommend reading these types of books to kids, which is now an "evidence-based practice," even though they also know it will "harm" a smaller group of kids by making them eat fewer veggies.

The next time you hear "the research says" or "this is an evidence-based practice," keep this example in mind. Your child might fall into the group that eats more carrots after reading a story about a carrot-loving bunny, but they also might not change or even eat fewer carrots than ever. The only way to know whether stories help your child eat better is to get curious, try it, and pay attention to what happens. And when you see a study cited that says, "If you do *x*, *y*, or *z*, *something specific* will happen to your child," take it with a grain of salt. There's no way anyone else knows what will work best for your child.

MAKING ROOM FOR RESEARCH

Sometimes, experimental research can't be conducted on important topics because of concerns about ethics or the health risks to participants. For example, it would be unethical to enroll children in an experimental study on the effects of cannabis edibles on childhood development. Observational studies are hugely important in these cases, and when enough high-quality observational studies are conducted, scientists can use them to establish causality. Public health recommendations—such as the recommendation to quit smoking, or to decrease intake of processed meat—are largely built on observational studies and yet have been used to establish that smoking and processed meats can cause cancer. As an example, more than eight hundred studies were reviewed to determine if red meat or processed meats *cause* cancer. Four hundred of those studies addressed processed meat, and it was found to be carcinogenic; seven hundred studies addressed red meat, and it was found to probably be carcinogenic; but there wasn't enough data to strongly determine causality. However, observational studies can also be fodder for headlines like "Lead and Cadmium Found in Sweet Potatoes and Carrots" or "Parents Slammed for Using TV in the Latest Vegetable Study." When I talk about the results of observational studies in this book, I will generally say "researchers *observed*" or "*x* is *associated* with *y*," to help make it clear when research is observational and cannot explain the cause.

Even at its best—meaning there are multiple well-designed studies with similar findings—research can never give us all the answers. First, it's incredibly rare for any study to show that all the people in a study had the same outcome. Usually, there is a combination of different results—some people experience a positive change, other people experience no change or a negative change. Additionally, sometimes how *much* change people experience isn't very meaningful. Let's say most of the kids in the carrot experiment were eating five carrots per snack and then, after hearing the story about carrots, they ate ten carrots per snack—that's a meaningful difference. But if the kids ate only one bite more after they heard the story, for a total of five carrots and one bite, that's not inspiring. It might still be true that "most kids ate more carrots," but one bite more isn't "meaningful." This difference is called the *effect size*, and most child feeding studies report small effect sizes, so that's something to consider as you change your behavior based on "the research."

Another limitation of research is that it only answers the questions that it asks. In the case of books and veggies, the question was "Do preschoolers who read fun books about veggies eat more veggies?" It didn't ask about why the parent was reading books or who chose the books. Maybe the parents who read fun books about fruits and veggies are better at cooking. And if researchers suspect that, they will need to ask new questions. Just by changing the questions, what the research shows can change dramatically. The recommendation may change from "read fun books about veggies to your child" to "learn to cook delicious veggies."

One final limitation to keep in mind when considering feeding research: It often fails to consider all the different types of kids out there. It might exclude kids of certain races or ethnicities, or kids who are neurodivergent. Research in child feeding is often conducted with white, middle-to-upper-class children and their mothers. If your child is neurodivergent, has a medical condition, lives in a community with cultural practices that are different from most communities, is a racial minority, or has only one parent, the research may not even apply. Fathers are often not included in child feeding research, even though studies observe fathers and mothers answer surveys about their children and child feeding differently and have different relationships with their children. It's possible that if data was gathered from all parents, the conclusions of studies would be completely different.

There are also all sorts of differences between kids that aren't as obvious to researchers as race or gender, which means researchers don't always think to study these factors, or they study them from only one angle. For example, researchers have commonly assumed certain strategies parents use, like using food to soothe or pushing kids to eat food, resulted in their child eating poorly and thus are unhelpful. They also commonly assumed that other parental strategies, like structured and supportive feeding, resulted in their child eating healthfully. What they may not have considered was that the parents using those "unhelpful" strategies often had children with "difficult" temperaments (negative, withdrawn, and not very adaptable), and so mealtimes with those kids were more stressful and they needed to adapt. Naturally, these parents would start using different and perhaps more coercive feeding strategies if their child was difficult at mealtimes. On the other hand, if a child can self-regulate, is easy to feed, and thus their parent is less stressed, they will feel more confident using more commonly recommended structured practices. Researchers also may not have considered whether a parent's feeding choices are a response to their child's innate eating style, such as loving to eat, having difficulty managing their emotions, or being impulsive. It's easily just as true that a child who loves eating from day one may lead a parent to restrict food, but we don't have much research data on this. And that creates uncertainty about the parent feeding practices that we recommend right now. Perhaps we should be using different parenting practices based on a child's temperament.

WHEN CURIOSITY OUTPERFORMS RESEARCH

With media sources, specialists, and influencers passionately promoting conflicting "research" outcomes, it's no surprise that many parents are left wondering what's right for their child. Should they limit cookies or let their kids eat whatever they want? Should they enforce a "one-bite rule" or let their child decide how much to eat at mealtime? This is another example of where eating with curiosity becomes essential. While there is more conclusive evidence in fields such as medicine, child feeding research does not provide the kind of certainty we would ideally like to have on most aspects of child feeding. There are so many factors affecting how a child will respond to different food practices, which means "the research" cannot always tell you what is right for your child. It can give suggestions or a starting place or provide observations about other kids and other families, but only *you* can see what is happening in your family. Curiosity, coupled with the other practical strategies throughout this book, will help you navigate the shifting recommendations and the unique needs of your individual family to make the best possible choices for feeding your child.

Over the years, many people have reached out to tell me that my social media content has helped them. They tried some of the strategies I suggested in a video, and their child's eating improved or their stress levels went down. Great! But there are always parents for whom the strategies didn't work, even when followed to a T. That's because all kids are different. It's also why curiosity is now my favorite parenting practice. Curiosity gives you permission to break the "rules" if they aren't working for your family. As long as we remain curious about why something isn't working, and what might work instead, we're doing what we need to do.

To dial into your curiosity, start by considering your child's personality, temperament, eating traits, and other personal qualities. Did you win the "easy to feed" kid lottery? Then the latest evidence-based suggestions (plus a hefty side of broccoli) may be all you need. Is your child failing to gain weight as expected? Then you might choose what to feed them based on what they are willing to eat rather than the recommendations of specific research. Does your child value their autonomy and push back against your suggestions? That might mean you have to be extra careful about avoiding pressure or praise.

You'll also want to think about who *you* are. Do you struggle in your relationship with food? If so, you might use parenting practices that help prioritize your mental health. Does food waste or your child complaining about a meal make you lose it? Maybe a quick breathing practice while you're prepping the meals could help you come to the table more calmly. There might even be a practice that is largely supported by research conclusions, such as the benefit of family meals, but based on your life circumstances, this practice is just not doable for your family. The research may point to the benefits of family meals for child development, but that research is not specific to your child. Don't waste time and energy worrying about negative consequences when a practice does not work for your family. Instead, remind yourself that if and when you *can* do the best practice, you will, and if you encounter a challenge before that, you have what it takes to handle it. Until then, don't stress about it. Move on to a strategy that is achievable for your family.

Next, hang on to your common sense. Let's imagine that someone you trust says, "The evidence-based recommendation is that you should never limit any foods you offer your child." Then let's say that you have a bag of prunes stored in a place that your toddler, who absolutely loves prunes, can easily reach. I don't care how much you trust the person who told you never to limit the foods you offer your child. You need to listen to *your* common sense (which I hope will tell you that limiting the number of prunes your toddler is allowed to eat is better for everyone than changing stinky diapers all night). Your common sense will also come in handy if a "best practice" could have a negative impact on you or your children. For example, if your child routinely eats so much that they vomit because they can't recognize when they are full, common sense should tell you that serving unlimited portions may not be a good strategy in your home.

At the same time, it's important to recognize that some of the customs or "rules" that have shaped our common sense aren't doing us any favors. For example, many adults have told me they find themselves eating beyond when they are full because as kids, they were told that it was important to "clean their plates." In this case, with our kids, we want to revise the belief that underlies this piece of common sense, allowing our kids to stop eating when they feel full. Or maybe what we believe is a common-sense understanding is actually based on messaging generated by the food or wellness industries. For example, the wellness industry has been spreading the message for decades that many, if not all, children have hidden micronutrient deficiencies and need a daily multivitamin. The message is so common that giving a child a multivitamin has become conventional wisdom to many people. The reality is that while multivitamins have a place, not all children need supplements and for those that do, a multivitamin may not be the right answer—a more common-sense approach might be to find out if your child has deficiencies or inadequate nutrient intake first, then to decide which supplement will solve their problem. If you're facing a feeding struggle with your child, it may be a sign that it's time to try a new strategy. That might involve consulting a specialist, trying something that worked for a friend with their kids, or coming up with your own strategy.

Eating with curiosity involves being willing to experiment and facing a certain degree of uncertainty. This can feel uncomfortable, but it's incredibly important. Maintaining an experimental attitude keeps your options open. Consider, for example, feeding an infant. If you've heard that breastfeeding is the evidence-based best practice and it's something that seems achievable for you, you could start with the mindset that breastfeeding your baby will be an experiment. If the experiment yields positive results for you and everyone is doing well (your baby is gaining weight and you are not physically or mentally suffering from the task), then your experiment showed breastfeeding was a good fit for you. However, if your baby is unable to latch and not getting the nourishment they need, and you are at your wit's end, then the experiment showed that breastfeeding is not a good fit for you, and the best thing for your child is to try a different feeding option. Experiments that end in "This was not at all helpful for us" are just as successful as those that end in "Wow, this is great for us!"

Research often doesn't acknowledge another core reason for our choices in what and how we feed our children—our identity. Food brings people together in a way that few things can. Food represents celebration, ritual, and connection. It signals who we are and who we are not. Many religions have long-standing food traditions that create a strong sense of belonging and meaning. More recently, certain food lifestyles have become important pieces of people's identities. Practices such as "plant-based" eating and "clean eating," to name a few, can provide a significant sense of identity to those who follow them, with specific foods signaling whether people are in or out of the group. Some groups might have "mascot foods" that they rally around, and whether a person eats them or not might signal whether that person is in a group or not. Examples include seed oils, animal-based foods, pork, grains, foods with artificial food dyes, or "bulletproof" coffee.

There's nothing wrong with forming a sense of belonging around shared beliefs, opinions, or values, or having certain foods or dietary lifestyles as flags to rally around. And we must think about what we're doing with that sense of belonging. Holding certain food beliefs doesn't necessarily mean we're right or that those beliefs are good for everyone—and we shouldn't shame or attack others who hold different beliefs. Sometimes people who provide information about mascot foods, especially trending ones, pick and choose which research studies they will talk about, rather than looking at a whole research bucket. This is why we need curiosity. If people are spreading information about food, those who are listening to that content need to be curious and ask themselves *why* this information is being shared. Because it's evidence-based and important? Or because it upholds one specific identity or perspective? If you feel very defensive or the need to criticize someone based on their opinion about a food, it might signal that the food is a symbol of your identity.

HOW OVER *WHAT*

A word of warning: Sometimes when we lead with curiosity, we end up with more dilemmas and fewer black-and-white answers. This is especially true when the "best practice" du jour is not working for your child, and your only other option is something that goes against "the research." This is why, throughout this book, I emphasize the *how* of feeding our kids over the *what*. In a world where we're constantly bombarded by information, opinions, and recommendations, it's often unclear *what* we are supposed to do. And overall, child feeding research supports the idea that there isn't always one right thing to do. Something we do have control over, however, is *how* we do whatever it is that we do. *How* we approach the task of feeding our children and eating together will always make a difference.

When it comes to feeding our children, it's important to get in touch with our core values. Regardless of the feeding approach we take, our connection with our kids matters most of all. Honoring that connection is a core value. We also want our kids to understand that they have worth and dignity as they are *today*, regardless of their body size, shape, or health status. Honoring self-worth is another core value. When we commit to honoring these core values, rather than insisting that our kids need to eat a certain number of vegetables a day or have a certain BMI, we emphasize the *how* over the *what*, and we are able to take a more thoughtful approach to feeding.

Let's say, for example, that your child has been diagnosed with a health condition for which they specifically need to start eating more greens. They don't like greens yet, so you will need to embrace an experimenter's mindset to get your child on board. You decide that you will start requiring them to try a bite of greens at dinner, but you recognize that it's a totally different experience for your child to hear you sternly say, "Eat those greens or you'll be sitting here all night!" versus cheerily saying, "We're all going to take a bite of our greens together—three, two, one, go!" In this case, we know that our kid needs to start eating greens, but it's *how* we approach this challenge that will have the greatest impact on their body and their relationship with us. They may have to try a food they detest, but at least they will know that you and the rest of the family are in their corner. The *how* involves getting everyone to eat their greens together, using a warm or playful tone, using confident and caring body language, and keeping calm when things get tricky. It also involves listening to your kid and their experience. For a child, learning to eat greens when they don't like them isn't exactly fun. Let them tell you that. Listen, keep your cool, and let them know that you get it.

How over *what* doesn't mean that you sit back and let your child take charge. You can be supportive of your child while also being firm about continuing with a change. In the greens scenario, you can empathize with your child's plight while holding firm that everyone will continue to take a bite every night. This may feel uncomfortable. Good strategies and good experiments don't always give us the warm fuzzies or make everyone happy. It may also be a real headache to have everyone in the family take a bite of greens together every night. However, if we give the experiment a good shot, we may start to see that everyone in the family is starting to try those greens with less complaining. Eventually, the headache lessens, we keep going, and we start to observe that our health needs are being met, and it was worth making the change for the family. But it was the *how* that got you there.

At the end of the day, I would love to have a definitive answer to every food-related question, and it would be great if "the research" could always provide that. It would make my job—and yours—a lot easier. But it's important to recognize and accept that this level of certainty on the research just isn't possible. Even within one family, our approach will need to change as our family members change. The one thing we *can* be certain of? As parents, the best way forward is to listen to our kids and to remain curious to determine what works for the whole family. This might mean paying attention to a breakdown of the latest peer-reviewed published research consensus and trying out new recommendations, or it might involve using our own creativity to find a solution unique to our situation. It will definitely mean interpreting the research through the filter of your specific family and your specific needs. Eating with curiosity gives parents—and kids—the courage and flexibility to keep moving forward, even when we face challenges. In the end, the lack of definitive answers may be a gift that enables us to cultivate curiosity and flexibility in our kids, so that as they grow, they become curious about their own health and feel empowered to experiment and eat what works for them.

2

EAT WITH EMBODIED INDEPENDENCE

One morning, when my son was five, I decided to make smoothies for breakfast. I was on a smoothie kick, and the kids were mostly enjoying it. But on this morning, I tried adding a new, supposedly tasteless, protein powder to our smoothies, and I gave one to my son to drink.

"Yuck!" he said.

"You haven't even tried it," I pointed out.

"I did. It tastes like sand."

"You need to drink it!" I insisted.

"It tastes like sand. I'm not going to drink it!"

By now, I was ramped up and pushing the glass into his hand. "How are you supposed to make it through the day if you don't eat your breakfast?! You have to drink it. You have to drink it and drink all of it!"

Eyes wide, he took a sip and then quickly slipped out the door to head to school.

Once he was gone, I sat there in the kitchen, feeling surprised over the way things had gone sideways. My job is to tell parents *not* to force their kids to eat, but the words had come tumbling out of my mouth in a moment where I was feeling stressed and worried about how much he was eating. I wanted him to understand how important food is for his body. Also, although my son clearly didn't enjoy the drink, he did seem to enjoy my response. He seemed to be thinking, *Huh, that's new! I can make Mommy get worked up!* In the end, he had taken only a sip of the smoothie, which meant nothing to his daily nutrition.

Later, when I tried to drink his leftover smoothie so that it wouldn't be wasted, it tasted like . . . sand. I had to pour it down the drain. The cherry on top was that for the next two weeks, he rejected every smoothie I made to see if he could get me to repeat my performance. Life would have been a lot easier for both of us if I had just let him listen to his body.

As parents, we want our kids to have that solid breakfast before school, along with everything else they need to thrive. We also want them to be able to make healthy choices for themselves when we're not there. As they grow up, we want them to know how to plan, prep, and cook a variety of foods for themselves, we want them to be able to navigate food-related social situations, and we want them to know how to shop for groceries and balance a food budget. We also know all of this is difficult in today's food environment, where it can be challenging to consume a diet that provides their bodies with what they need to thrive.

This brings us to the second pillar of our program: eating with embodied independence, which we discussed briefly in the introduction. We need our kids to do more than just independently take care of their health. Embodied independence is about teaching them to live in and listen to their bodies, while helping them to understand what it means to intentionally nourish themselves.

The smoothie drama wasn't just about breakfast before school. It was about allowing my son the space to respond to what his body was telling him: "Dude, something about this smoothie doesn't taste right." In that moment of stress, he didn't have the space to listen to his body.

Teaching our kids to eat with embodied independence goes beyond equipping them with a basic understanding of nutrition so they can make healthy food choices. We also want them to have a good relationship with their bodies and with food. We don't want our kids skipping breakfast because they are afraid of gaining weight or because they dislike their bodies. We want to reduce their risk for disordered eating and internalized weight bias as much as we want to lower their risk of other diseases. We want them to fully live in their bodies, understanding how they feel at any given time and to be able to enjoy eating.

Embodiment is a wonky word, but it fits the bill here. An embodied child is positively connected to and experiencing their body. They feel their body sensations like fullness or thirst, as well as the heat of anger or the "butterflies" of anxiety. They can recognize, articulate, and respond to these feelings (also called *interoception*). Embodiment includes having an awareness of the connection between the way we feel in our physical bodies and how this is connected to our thoughts and emotions. This may sound like a tall order, especially for a kid, but you'd be surprised—especially if we nurture and encourage this skill early on. If you hear a school-age kid say something like "I feel nervous in my tummy," that's embodiment. Embodiment also describes what happens when a person tunes in to others and empathizes with them, such as when someone tears up when a friend cries.

Consider whether you've ever had a day like this: *Your mind was busy all day worrying or thinking about to-do lists, your child, or self-critical thoughts. You weren't happy with what you saw when you looked in the mirror that morning. When you got to the end of the day, you realized that you were ravenously hungry because you hadn't had enough to eat that day and that you also hadn't had enough water and were dehydrated. You generally felt unsettled, disconnected, and unhappy with how your body looked.* This describes the opposite of embodiment. It describes disconnection.

Now think about having a different kind of day: *You were engaged throughout the day and thought intentionally about what you were doing. You felt good about your purpose for the day and really appreciated what your body could do. You enjoyed eating, ate the amount that felt comfortable for you during meals, and you drank water when you were thirsty throughout the day. You felt connected and glad to be able to care for your body.* This is embodiment. It's living in your body and appreciating it. When we're embodied, we lovingly respond to and care for our physical selves. Embodiment also helps protect us from disordered eating.

A child or an adult who experiences embodiment eats when they are hungry, stops eating when they are satisfied, eats a variety of foods to meet their health needs, and enjoys indulgences. A child or an adult with disordered eating, on the other hand, may heavily restrict how much food they eat to control their weight, or they may use food to regulate their emotions. They may be unable to respond to their hunger or fullness cues, or they may compulsively eat or overeat. They may not be able to eat enough variety to meet their nutrient needs, or they may have "rules" about what they are and are not allowed to eat. In its most extreme form, disordered eating becomes a clinical eating disorder that puts a person's health or life at risk. Many of us are familiar with eating disorders like anorexia nervosa (restricting food and purging or overexercising), bulimia nervosa (binge eating and purging or overexercising), and binge eating disorder (binge eating with no purging or overexercising). Avoidant/restrictive food intake disorder (ARFID; the inability to meet nutritional needs as a result of anxiety related to eating, lack of appetite, or restricting based on the sensory qualities of food) is another common eating disorder.

In general, most people have a mix of healthy and disordered ways of interacting with food. For example, I may crash with some emotional support ice cream and potato chips now and then, overeat during a holiday, or neglect to eat when I am very busy and didn't leave time to feed myself. These are all technically disordered eating behaviors, but they aren't representative of the way I eat regularly, and they aren't damaging my health or interfering with my day-to-day life. This is different from struggling with a clinical eating disorder that is ongoing, compromising our health, and interfering with everyday life.

When someone struggles with a clinical eating disorder, there are several factors that might have led to it. Kids who have a lot of exposure to the "thin ideal" are more likely to have eating disorders. Genetics, the gut microbiome, autoimmune diseases, parental influence, personality, physical development, and mental health conditions are also factors associated with disordered eating. Researchers are still learning about the causes of disordered eating, but one thing we do know is that when we encourage embodied eating in our kids, it helps to protect their relationship with their bodies and with food.

PUSHING BACK ON THE THIN IDEAL

Given the food environment that surrounds us, which includes exposure to diet culture, food marketing, the thin ideal, and more, teaching embodied independence is tricky. But it starts with becoming aware of our own internalized weight bias. Children need to be taught that their bodies are worthy of love, respect, and care, regardless of shape and size or how they change over time, and they need to hear this from adults who really believe what they are saying. It's important to reinforce the message with kids that a person's worth is not determined by their body size. We want to encourage our kids to make food choices based on what their bodies need rather than based on external standards of what someone "should" eat or look like. Parents need to be intentional about cultivating this mindset and especially diligent regarding kids' exposure to the thin ideal.

When I was growing up, I was not allowed to buy teen or beauty magazines. I don't remember what explanation my parents gave me for this rule, but whatever it was, I didn't push back very much. Once I got older and moved out of the house, I continued to avoid these magazines. The messages and images in them just didn't sit right with me, because on some level, I knew they weren't healthy for me. My parents couldn't eliminate my exposure to the thin ideal, but this one rule reduced it, and it had a lasting effect.

Media is one of the biggest drivers of body dissatisfaction for children. The more that we can do as parents to reduce our children's exposure to media outlets that normalize disordered eating and the thin ideal, from TV shows to social media accounts promoting thinness to apps that alter appearance to AI conversations on weight loss, the better. Food, calorie, and fitness trackers can also be problematic, even when they appear harmless or even healthy. The thin ideal can work itself into any topic, but industries that commonly benefit by maintaining the thin ideal include beauty, fashion, weight loss, fitness, wellness, "lifestyle," and nutrition. Obviously, these categories are not dangerous across the board, but if your kid is very interested in one of these areas, it's worth paying attention. Also, beware of any media source or app that "serves up" content to you or your child that you didn't ask for with features such as "watch next," "you may be interested in," "explore," and "for you."

These platforms take user behavior and manipulate it to give us more of what they "think" we are interested in to keep us using the app or media source. This could mean, for example, that if based on your child's age, gender, or other information, the app suggests a "thinspiration" or bodybuilding video, and your child watches it out of curiosity, the app will then send them more thinspiration or bodybuilding content. Developers of these technologies know that if something is novel, shocking, or exciting, people will keep watching. A child can start by watching a YouTube video about how to make a smoothie, then progressively find themselves watching a video about the health benefits of smoothies, then smoothies for weight loss, then healthy ways to lose weight, then unhealthy ways to lose weight, and then pro–anorexia nervosa content—all without having ever searched for anything related to anorexia nervosa.

At the end of the day, every family will have to work out what reduced exposure looks like for them, whether this means prohibiting a magazine or TV show or app outright, or allowing only selective or supervised access. This probably won't be fun. My kids haven't given my husband and me a hug and thanked us when we've said no to a popular video game or movie, even if it was accompanied by a yes to another one. Setting a boundary around media use often takes courage. You can do it, though, even if it's uncomfortable. Another crucial piece of this is working to build your child's media literacy skills, which can start as early as preschool or kindergarten. This includes teaching them to evaluate information presented in media outlets, to think critically about it, and to become conscious consumers and creators of media.

As a parent, you can do this by explaining to your kids how images in various forms of media, such as food commercials, are manipulated to sell products—that shiny spray is used to make food look fresh and juicy, or that kids cannot suddenly flip upside down on skateboards after they eat a certain kind of cereal. Kids also need to know that this also applies to media their friends create or that people upload—the acne was photoshopped out, skin folds smoothed over, and body size changed. In our house, my husband and I help promote this skill by asking questions to promote critical thinking. For example, with the cereal commercial, we might ask the kids one or two of the following questions:

"Who do you think made this ad?"

"Why did they make it?"

"What is their opinion?"

"Is what we're seeing real?"

"What do the people who made this commercial want you to believe/feel/do after seeing this?"

"What did you see that gave you clues to answer these questions?"

I've recently noticed my own kids utilizing their media literacy skills during family movie nights. They've become obsessed with special effects and figuring out what is real and what is fake, so watching a live-action movie involves a barrage of commentary like, "Is that computer generated?" or "I bet they had a stunt double for that flying move." It's not my favorite phase (sometimes I just want to watch a movie without having a side discussion), but the ability to discern what's real from what's not is an incredibly important life skill.

Along with the thin ideal, the weight-loss, health insurance, and food industries (as well as plenty others) promote the ideology that individuals are solely responsible for all elements of their health and wellness, including their weight. This idea of sole personal responsibility for health is a great business tool. It allows companies to make promises about their programs, supplements, or foods to convince us to buy in, but if something goes wrong, they can blame *us*—not their marketing, bogus products, hyperpalatability, or the food environment they've created. We're accused of poor choices or lack of willpower, or led to believe something is inherently wrong with us. However, there is ample research demonstrating that weight and wellness are determined by a variety of factors, many of which we may have little or no control over, such as our genetics, socioeconomic status, food security, and environment. However, the emphasis on personal responsibility gets food companies off the hook for the public health problems they create, even if research tells us that food marketing overrides our ability to choose. This also perpetuates internalized bias and weight stigma. When we shift our perspective and acknowledge that weight is influenced by many factors—and teach our kids the same—internalized weight bias and judgment can decrease. Your child will feel it. It will make a difference.

As parents, we can do our part to stop perpetuating the thin ideal at home. When we talk about our bodies or the bodies of others as being the wrong size, or say that we need to change them or lose weight, children internalize the idea that certain-size bodies are bad. A parent openly dieting or having negative weight bias is one of the largest risk factors for internalized weight bias and body dissatisfaction in children. This means that if parents discuss their own weight-loss journeys, their child is more likely to be unhappy with their body and want to diet, too. I can't overstate how important it is to avoid exposing your child to adult weight-loss talk, especially if you are the one pursuing weight loss (seriously, keep the bathroom scale in the closet so they don't see it). Talking about your child's body can be equally harmful. Even saying something that seems positive like, "You're nice and slim," or "You're the perfect weight," reinforces the idea that certain-size bodies are bad. Don't mention your thoughts on your child's body size or shape. In fact, unless you are discussing weight in a practical sense, such as "You weigh thirty pounds, so you need this many medicine tablets," or your child brings is up, avoid discussing body shapes and sizes—period. If other adults in your child's life, such as relatives or babysitters, are talking about weight or body size, you may need to have a conversation with them about avoiding this topic when your child is around.

Avoiding weight talk doesn't mean you need to avoid talking about health. When we make our child's overall health the focus instead of weight, we give them a more embodied perspective of it. That means that rather than saying, "We eat a lot of veggies so we can stay thin," you might say, "We eat a lot of veggies to have a healthier heart," or, "These veggies make me feel stronger." With this simple shift, diet and lifestyle changes like eating more veggies or getting more exercise become a way of caring for our bodies instead of a way of changing how we look.

Finally, even if you struggle to reduce your child's exposure to the thin ideal, just by teaching them that the thin ideal exists, you are helping protect them. Most successful eating disorder prevention programs include teaching children to be aware of the thin ideal and to recognize it as unattainable and stigmatizing. Whatever your child's size, they need to understand the dangers of weight stigma and the thin ideal. I like the term *weightism*, which describes language or behavior that promotes weight stigma, because it sounds like *racism*, which is a term kids should be familiar with and know is very wrong.

When my kids started going to friends' houses and watching movies and borrowing books, I started using the resources from Common Sense Media to find out if those movies and books contained weightism, racial stereotypes, and branded product placements. When my kids watched *The Goonies*, a movie from the '80s that I had forgotten the details of, I checked the review and saw that there was quite a bit of weight-based stereotyping in it. So, when I had a chance, I chatted with them about what they noticed about how the heavier character was portrayed and how this contributes to weight stigma. These days, I point out weight stigma and the thin ideal in the same way I would if we came across racism while reading, watching, or listening to something together. I might say something like, "I could have done without them making a big deal about how the character had gained weight. Weight stigma!" "They made that person look thinner than they are . . ." or "They are showing that only thin people won the competition. I wonder why." It's also something that may come up in their interactions with friends. Kids need to be able to recognize it.

INTEROCEPTION AND PREDICTABLE PARENTING

A core element of embodiment is *interoception*, which is the term for being able to recognize what your body is experiencing—such as when you're hungry, full, cold, hot, sad, happy, anxious, worried, embarrassed, or if you have to pee. It is important for a child to develop a sense of interoception so that they can take care of their body, tolerate what they feel, and respond appropriately. Interoception is a sense that often needs training throughout life to be used effectively. For example, adults may be good at knowing when they are hungry, full, or cold, but may have to learn to identify specific emotions like anger or sadness if they weren't taught how as children. Some children easily learn to identify hunger, fullness, and other body signals, while others need more deliberate teaching and training. They may confuse feelings of hunger with feelings of boredom, for example, or not recognize when they are hungry. The development of interoception can be affected by developmental delays, sensory processing issues, neurodivergence, mental health conditions, and their environment.

We can teach kids to use their interoceptive sense in the same ways we teach other skills, by modeling and giving them opportunities to practice. By talking about how *you* feel or helping your child talk about how they feel, you provide opportunities to learn. You can narrate your own experience—"I feel hot. Some ice will cool me down"—or, one I used with my kids: "My middle feels all squiggly. That means I'm feeling anxious." Feeding your child offers daily opportunities to help them develop their interoception and trust it. When you provide meals, you might say, "You don't have to eat if you're not hungry," "You don't have to finish your plate. We'll save that for later," or "Only you know if your tummy is empty or full." Phrases like these teach kids to listen to their feelings of hunger and fullness and respond to them. Of course, you may worry that if you focus on interoception, your child will eat three bites of dinner and then be hungry right before bedtime—because you've seen that happen. That's why embodiment alone isn't the full pillar. We also need independence—the ability to make the right decision for our bodies using the information in our minds. A great way to teach this independence piece is with a practice that I call *predictable parenting*.

When you use predictable parenting, your child knows what to expect, consistently, when it comes to eating in your home. They know when dinner is coming, and they know what the mealtime rules are in your home. Predictable parenting will give your children the tools to feed themselves independently over time. With this approach, you get to create the "food environment" in your home, one that will model and teach your child what independence could look like for them once they are making decisions about what to eat on their own. At the start, you will take care of all the eating logistics in your home, from the food on the plates to the time dinner is served. Eventually, you want your kids to have the know-how to do this for themselves. Think of this as running the Eating with Independence restaurant in your home.

Let's think about restaurants for a minute. When we go out to eat at a restaurant, we know what to expect. We know the rules and customs, what's on the menu, and when lunch or dinner starts. We might not love everything about the restaurant, we may be annoyed that we always have to put our napkins on our laps or that they always put ice in the water, but we go along with it. Similarly, your child may not always be happy with your boundaries, whether those are around the timing of dinner or the food offerings or something entirely different. In fact, you might as well expect, right now, that your child often will be unhappy with your boundaries (I probably didn't have to tell you that). This doesn't mean you're doing anything wrong or that you're ruining your child's relationship with food, however. It means that your child is expressing their feelings and learning to eat with independence.

As the parents and the owners of the Eating with Independence restaurant, one of your jobs is to decide the menu. Your restaurant isn't a diner. You absolutely do not have to be a short-order cook. It's more like a fancy restaurant that has a fixed menu decided by the chef. While you may get a choice of one or two things, the choices are limited. As a parent, you can feel confident saying, "This is what's for dinner." Hard stop. Unless your child has a health concern, the more consistently and firmly you hold this boundary, the better.

I won't sugarcoat the fact that holding your "restaurant boundaries" can be unpleasant (to put it mildly). A few years ago, I served rice and chicken stir-fry for dinner, and my son told us he didn't want it—he wanted yogurt and a cheese stick instead. Getting up and getting a different dinner isn't part of our restaurant, and my son and I ended up in a heated back-and-forth, as he demanded to know why he couldn't have that yogurt and cheese stick. Eventually, I blurted out, "Research suggests that parents who get up and get kids a second meal have kids who are more likely to determine what is served, eat less variety, and have reduced diet quality. Plus, it's stressful for the family."

"How do you know?" he came back.

My husband chimed in, "This is her specialty."

With visions of spending the next hour in front of my laptop, I grumbled, "I can provide the research references if you would like."

I fully respect a person who wants to see the receipts, even if they're only eight, so I would have followed through on my references offer. On that day, though, I was off the hook. He was actually satisfied with my why. He stopped asking questions, ate some rice, and filled up later at bedtime snack (which is part of our predetermined eating routine). It helped that we have a track record of holding firm on this boundary. This sort of back-and-forth about what's for dinner is uncommon. He knows the drill. We're predictable.

Holding firm regarding your menu will ultimately show your kids what balanced eating looks like. While a preschooler might choose mac and cheese every night because that's what they can think of, that's not a balanced diet. You may choose to serve mac and cheese sometimes (or a lot), but you will also serve a variety of other foods over time. Exposing children to a variety of foods—and modeling eating them—teaches kids to eat different foods and minimizes picky eating, which helps them take care of their bodies. It also teaches them how to put together balanced meals. These are both essential parts of eating independence.

From my perspective as a parent and professional, the stronger and more predictable you can be about your restaurant boundaries (regardless of your child's emotions in the moment), the more in touch with their body your child will be, the more variety they will eat, and the less they will push back. As you're approaching a meal, rather than asking your child, "What do you want for dinner?" lean into the *how* and focus on connecting with them. You might say something like, "I'm looking forward to having dinner with you."

There is one important ground rule, though. The meals you offer must have at least one food that your child is comfortable with. If I visited a restaurant that only served dishes I hadn't learned to like yet, such as fried liver, raw onions, and sautéed mushrooms, I would leave the restaurant hungry. If the restaurant also served bread and butter on the side, however, I would still be annoyed, but at least I could eat some bread and not leave hungry. Plus, if I took the edge off my hunger with the bread, I might have more capacity to try a bite of fried liver and see what a mushroom tasted like on my bread. I might learn I like mushrooms now.

This approach will look different at different stages with your child as they go from complete inability to make choices in infancy, to being able to choose between two options you've given them, to helping you plan the menu. You decide how much choice they get, and it will vary based on your child's needs. For example, if your child is older, you may allow them to choose their own afternoon snack from a snack cabinet, but you are still choosing what goes in the cabinet. You're also the owner of the restaurant. If you want to always have a second meal option like peanut butter and jelly, that's fine, as long as you're predictable about it.

Whatever the menu looks like in your house, you also get to decide your restaurant's "ambiance"—this can help develop your child's interoception. For example, distractions such as screens usually make it harder for kids to tune in and feel their hunger and fullness cues, and reducing them can help kids respond to their bodies.

Sitting is also important—for safety as well as learning to eat mindfully and paying attention to the way that food makes them feel. If you've got an active toddler, they may only be able to sit for a few minutes. You can start with a small number of minutes and slowly work them up to a longer time. If your child is sitting with their feet on a rest or the floor and their elbows can be at a ninety-degree angle to the table (your teacher was right; one day you *would* need geometry in real life), you'd be amazed at how much better they will eat.

Interoception can also be developed by helping make a child's hunger and fullness feelings "louder" with boundaries like *when* meals and snacks are served. Think of it as setting your restaurant's "hours." You'll provide food routinely so that your child knows you're a predictable source of nourishment and care. If you put boundaries around snacks and mealtimes, your kids will come to the table hungry enough to feel their hunger and their fullness cues clearly. Your routine around snacks and mealtimes could be grounded in a set schedule like they do in day care, school, camps, and some work settings. Or it could be more flexible, where food is incorporated into the daily flow of activities. You could also use "eating windows," where a child can choose when to eat their snack within a certain period of time. It could be that meals are scheduled, but snacks are provided on an "as-needed" basis when you decide they are needed. You can set your restaurant's hours however you want, as long as they're predictable.

Keep in mind that snacks throughout the day are not mandatory. Yes, it's the cultural norm in the US right now to feed kids lots of snacks, but consider that in 1977, children ages two through six ate about 1.3 snacks per day, and children seven through twelve ate about 1.2 snacks per day. By 2014, in the United States, the average two-to-five-year-old ate about 3 snacks per day, and children six through eleven years old ate about 2.5 snacks per day. Biologically, most humans, especially once they are out of early childhood (older than age five or so), do not *need* snacks. In fact, frequent eating, "grazing," or "snacking" is associated with lower diet quality, cavities, and children being less able to listen to their hunger and fullness cues. The cultural phenomenon of snacking has actually decreased children's diet quality.

I'm not suggesting you stop feeding your child snacks if that's part of your routine. As I said, it's our cultural norm. Three snacks a day are a formal part of my family's routine. You and I know, however, that if our kids eat a granola bar and bowl of crackers thirty-five minutes before dinner, they may pick at dinner, not feel like eating the veggies, or decide they don't want to eat at all (and then be hungry as soon as you tell them it's time to brush their teeth). Those hunger cues are important. The key to hunger cues is giving kids time to get hungry by having times when you don't serve food (usually several hours between meals). It helps kids "hear" their hunger and eat better and more fully at meals, which in turn helps them hear their fullness. Allowing your child to experience the feeling of being reasonably hungry is important for their health, their interoception, and their trust in you as a loving caregiver who provides food in a predictable way. While there may be exceptions, especially for children who have certain medical conditions or have experienced food insecurity, learning to read hunger cues is a core component of eating with embodied independence for the majority of children.

Parents frequently ask me, "What do you do when your child chooses not to eat a meal and then asks for a snack before your usual snack time?" Think about when you had a young toddler. You went grocery shopping with them, with a plan to be back before their afternoon nap. They usually slept about two hours in the afternoon, unless they slept for fifteen minutes in the car before a nap! If that happened, they'd probably wake up when you took them into the house and then wouldn't go down for their regular nap. Then they were fussy for the rest of the day. So, what did you do if you were driving home before the afternoon nap time? Whatever you could to keep them awake on the fifteen-minute drive home. You sang songs, rolled down the window, turned on the air conditioner. You talked and handed them a toy. Whatever it took. Then when you got them home, you properly put them down for a nap, and they slept for their normal two hours. The day was saved! Your child was responding to their biological need for sleep, and you provided the structure so that they could respond to their need in a way that allowed them to get everything they needed to be healthy.

It's similar with eating. If you have plentiful food resources in your home, you know your child has another meal or snack coming right around the corner. Assuming you are being kind and patient with your child, if they ask for a snack and it's not snack time, they will be fine physically and emotionally until the next eating opportunity. Just like it's okay to be thirsty, too hot, too cold, or to have to "hold it" until you get to a restroom, being hungry for a bit won't hurt a child's relationship with their body or their embodiment. Your child may be hungry on the way back from an event in the morning, but rather than giving them an additional snack that will ruin their appetite for lunch, you can help them make it to lunchtime. You can warmly tell your child, "We're going to eat lunch as soon as we get home!" This doesn't mean you should never go off your eating routine or never give your child an extra snack. Just be mindful of the eating routine and how it's affecting your child's ability to listen to their body. The goal isn't to be rigid; the goal is to be predictable.

If the idea of withholding snacks is not palatable to you, that's okay. Some parents will always want to respond to their child's hunger in the moment and have food options available, and that could be due to their own history of food trauma or food insecurity, treatment of disordered eating in the home, a specific need for the child, or another personal philosophical approach. If this is the case for you, then you can think strategically about how you will offer snacks. You can serve something light (lower in fat and protein) like fruit, veggies, or a few crackers so that your child will still have a chance of being hungry at the next meal. You can also plan a grazing-friendly menu of meals and snacks, making sure the snacks are nutritious so that if they crowd out eating at meals, your child is still getting what they need.

THE RESTRICTION DEBATES

There are all sorts of reasons why a parent might choose to restrict what their child is eating—including allergies, medical conditions, food sensitivities, prevention of future health problems, the cost of certain foods, or religious beliefs.

Many parents choose to restrict hyperpalatable foods for the reasons we've discussed already—because they crowd out other nutrient-dense foods, they are associated with lower overall diet quality, and they make it harder to listen to our bodies and hunger cues.

As parents, we hear a lot of mixed messages about food restriction. We hear that we should be teaching our children about why some foods—like hyperpalatable foods, and those containing sugar, food dyes, contaminants, or processed ingredients—are bad for us, and that we should eliminate those foods from our kids' diets. At the same time, we also hear that restricting foods will cause disordered eating, will cause kids to become obsessed with the restricted foods, or will cause shame surrounding the restricted foods. We might also hear "moderation in everything." Which of these things is true? When it comes to restriction, parental confusion is understandable. Whether or not to restrict food, and how to implement restriction if you so choose, is a personal choice that you should make with your child's needs and your family's values in mind.

For a long time, I held the view that restricting foods was largely problematic for the reasons discussed above. However, after diving into the research for this book and digging into *hundreds* of studies, I made a surprising discovery: Research around child food restriction may be the most widely misrepresented research of any area of child feeding.

As it turns out, restriction likely doesn't have an impact on many children, and when and if it does, it likely has a small impact compared with other established factors affecting a child's eating habits, such as internalized weight bias, exposure to the thin ideal, and constant availability of hyperpalatable foods. There just isn't a lot of conclusive research on the effects of food restriction and there are very few experimental studies of restriction. In most of the studies that do exist, the researchers ask so few questions of parents that the results aren't practical or meaningful. (Were all sweet foods restricted or just some of them? Was the parent comforting when they told their child, "No more cookies today," or did they give the kid a guilt trip?) As a result, we can't apply this research to our lives. One group of researchers flat-out concluded that they see no evidence that restriction affects how kids eat in any way!

Accepting this conclusion, however, is difficult for many parents I talk to, because they've heard stories or read articles that claim they will damage their child's relationship with food by restricting. To help with that, here are the top six questions on the topic of restriction that I hear from parents, with the answers that I am able to provide based on what I would describe as a "responsible reading" of existing research (translation: thoroughly reading as many papers on the subject as possible and using lots of nuance!), and my recommendations for how to confront these challenges. I use cookies as the restricted food in question in examples below, but you can substitute in any hyperpalatable food that is relevant to you.

QUESTION #1

"*If I restrict cookies, will my child eat more cookies over time and fewer nutritious foods, reducing the amount of nutrition in their diet?*"

The simple answer is, "No one knows." It's unclear whether restriction correlates to diet quality. Some researchers have observed that restricted kids have more nutritious diets; others have observed that restricted kids have less nutritious diets. Based on the data available (or lack thereof), I would say that it's okay to practice curiosity and experiment with restricting versus not restricting the cookies to see whether your child eats a more or less nutritious diet as a result.

QUESTION #2

"*If I limited my child to two cookies whenever we have cookies, and then they get a chance to eat cookies at Grandma's house or at a birthday party, will they stuff themselves with cookies even if they are full from lunch? Will they become obsessed with cookies?*

Every child is different, and if they are obsessed with a certain hyperpalatable food, it likely won't be *because* you only let your child eat two of these food items. Let's examine this more closely. Some researchers have observed that restricted kids *aren't* more obsessed, and some have observed restricted kids *are* more obsessed. Some have even observed restricted kids being less obsessed *and* enjoying food more. Researchers think many factors, including genetics, temperament, age, and type and amount of restriction, may affect how a child responds to restriction. Even then, some researchers suspect the effect size (or the strength of the effect) of restriction may be so small it doesn't really matter. I think it's safe to say that if you restrict your child, they *may* eat extra cookies on a full stomach, and it is possible that restriction was part of the reason. It's probably more likely that your child would have always eaten extra cookies on a full stomach because they love cookies or because the cookies are hyperpalatable and it had little or nothing to do with whether you restricted them.

You might be wondering, "If restriction doesn't matter, why do I know a kid who makes a beeline for our candy dish when he comes over, because his mom doesn't keep candy at home?" It's a great question, and it seems like a lot of people have a story like this in their back pocket. These stories, however, generally don't consider factors like whether the child had an issue that caused the parent to restrict this food, or whether parents of kids who *aren't* obsessed with candy bowls were also restrictive. Just knowing that restriction is present isn't sufficient for understanding how kids react to food. We need a different paradigm for understanding this question. It's time for us to become familiar with the term *reactance.*

Psychological reactance theory suggests that people are motivated to take back their "freedom" if it's taken away or if they think it will be taken away. This is true as long as a person cares about the freedom and thinks they can get it back. According to this theory, when the individual does get the freedom back, they may go overboard in exercising this freedom, just because they can. If they don't care or if they don't think they can get it back, they'll move on. We can use this theory to guess what will happen to the child who's only allowed two cookies.

If a parent has only ever given their child two cookies from the time they started eating cookies and has calmly said no when they asked for more, and the child doesn't even know people eat more than two cookies, then reactance theory would suggest this child wouldn't have a strong motivation to take back their eating "freedom"—because the freedom they know is eating two cookies (assuming they don't have friends with different cookie-eating policies). It follows that if they have the chance to eat as much as they want, they might just eat two cookies and not think twice. Some kids may react differently, though. They may be more responsive to the hyperpalatable nature of the food and keep eating cookies just because they taste good and activate the brain's reward center.

Let's imagine the child, however, had always been allowed to eat as many cookies as they wanted, and the parent noticed the child was starting to eat more cookies each time they got the opportunity. It got to the point where the child would eat a whole box sometimes. It was affecting the child's health, so the parent implemented a rule of eating only two cookies. In that case, the child might feel their freedom had been removed, and if they went to someone's house with unlimited cookies just a week or two after the new "two-cookie rule," they may eat a whole box of cookies, hungry or not, just because they can. Their reactance has been triggered. They may continue to be obsessed with cookies if they think their parents will cave and start giving them unlimited cookies again. That's not the end of the story, though. According to reactance theory, as soon as the child realizes their parents *aren't* going to change the two-cookie rule, they will lose their motivation to care about cookies over time and move on. So it's possible the child may still be obsessed with cookies over time, but if so, it is much more likely to be because of the combination of the child's brain reward system, the hyperpalatable nature of the engineered cookies, or other physical or temperamental factors than whether the parents have a two-cookie rule.

Your child's reactance is important to pay attention to. If your child tends to overeat cookies because of their hyperpalatable nature and the way their brain is wired, setting limits early in childhood could potentially decrease their reactance. Contrary to the popular belief that "restriction" makes kids obsessed with food, for many kids, setting limits early on might mean less obsessing later.

If you're sitting slack-jawed, thinking, *But think of all the times you, Kids Eat in Color lady, said that restriction would surely make my kids obsessed with cookies and that I should be very careful about restricting them*, join the club. I'm sitting here thinking the same thing. My commitment to continuously studying research and re-evaluating recommendations involves the willingness to be flexible in the presence of new information, because it can lead to moments where I get to suggest a new framework for families. This is why the practice of curiosity is so foundational. We need that willingness to learn and try new things if what we have been trying isn't working. Letting go of some of the obsession with the effects of "restriction" and taking on the more useful framework of reactance is a change that will serve us well and is worth adjusting our thinking around.

QUESTION #3

"*If I always make cookies available from the time my kids are little, will that keep the cookies on a level playing field with other foods and prevent my child from developing an obsession with them?*"

Probably not. Let's use reactance theory to think through this scenario. The theory suggests that if a child has the freedom to eat unlimited cookies, they will have no reactance to push them to obsess over cookies, or to eat them beyond fullness and in the absence of hunger. However, in most cases, it is not possible to have unlimited access to an unlimited quantity of a food all the time. There will always be limitations of some kind on our access to foods. Most people have a certain amount of money for food (which might affect how many cookies they buy), they might have to make sure multiple people in the house get their fair share, and they are limited by things like seasonality, trips to the store, and what foods are in stock. Limits are normal. Having *limited* freedom is normal. Having *unlimited* freedom, on the other hand, is impossible, for all the reasons I just stated. So even if a child started out with unlimited access to cookies, they would encounter limits eventually, potentially triggering reactance.

Additionally, reactance is not the only thing that causes kids to get obsessed with something. Some kids just tend to obsess over things that excite them (like my child who became enamored with paper airplane making after he saw a demonstration at age three). Some kids react obsessively to hyperpalatable foods, some kids get obsessed with video games, some kids get obsessed with whatever their friends are obsessed with. So even in the case of a child who has always had complete cookie-eating freedom, they could still become obsessed with cookies.

If a child's temperament and brain chemistry don't lead to cookie obsession, why wouldn't a completely unrestricted approach be the best path to embodied independence? Wouldn't it teach them to regulate their eating better? I've heard from parents who offered their children unrestricted quantities of foods as toddlers, and these toddlers were able to self-regulate. Over time, however, many of these same parents reported that their kids stopped regulating well as they got older. Many of those same kids (I've seen it in my own kids, too) became more interested or even obsessed with various foods as they got more exposure, social hype, palate training, and time for hyperpalatable foods to adjust the reward systems in their brains. With all of this in mind, it's my hypothesis that giving kids unlimited access to all foods in early childhood makes embodied independence more difficult with hyperpalatable foods for many children. Reactance theory suggests that small limits from the start may preserve a child's sense of freedom *and* help them protect their sense of embodiment much more effectively than taking a restriction-free approach.

QUESTION #4

"If I limit my child to only two cookies in one sitting, will I cause them to have an eating disorder?"

The short answer to this question is, no, setting a two-cookie limit will not *cause* an eating disorder. Of all the risk factors for clinical eating disorders listed in research so far, having a parent who restricts food intake isn't among them. Most researchers studying restriction haven't generally observed that restricted kids have more disordered eating* or eating disorders.

At the same time, parents often tell me stories about how restrictive their own parents were and how much they believe it contributed to painful disordered eating for them later in life. Just like with the case of kids obsessed with candy dishes, it seems like there is a connection, but restriction itself may not be the actual problem.

Eating disorder studies suggest that there are *much* bigger risk factors than restriction at play when it comes to your child's relationship with food. For example, we know disordered eating can have a genetic component, and researchers have also observed that parents with more weight worries or disordered eating may be more likely to restrict, which suggests higher likelihood of genetics combined with other factors being the *cause*—a theory that is supported by research about eating disorders. Other factors, such as whether parents discuss their own or their child's body size and dieting, the child's personality traits and mental health, and their experience of the thin ideal, body dissatisfaction, food insecurity, or weight stigma also affect a child's risk of developing an eating

---

* Here I want to speak specifically to "disordered eating" in the sense of weight control, dieting, binge eating, and purging.

disorder. There's a tiny bit of research that suggests children whose caregivers use restrictive or critical messages may have guilt or shame related to eating and their bodies or in the future when they are grown up. This suggests *how* parents are restricting may play a role in disordered eating. The fixation, effort, and worry related to "restriction" in general distracts from these bigger issues.

Fearmongering messages like "Research says children will have disordered eating if they aren't allowed to eat as much candy as they want on holidays" are quite literally made up. An alternative message more accurate to the research is, "Some kids are more likely to have disordered eating, and if a parent has one of those kids, the parents might restrict how much candy they eat on holidays in response. For some kids, it may make their disordered eating worse; for other kids, it may make their eating better; for the rest, it may have no effect at all."

QUESTION #5

"If I don't let my child have cookies at all, will that make them more obsessed with cookies, because they are completely forbidden?"

The "forbidden fruit" effect is often brought up in conversations about restriction. The idea is that if you tell someone they aren't allowed to have something, they will want it. I think most of us have observed this firsthand in some capacity—a greater interest or fascination in something you aren't allowed to engage in.

As a child of the '80s, I spent my fair share of time pretending to be a movie star smoking my classic gum "cigarettes" (cigarette marketing to children, anyone?). I was curious about smoking, so at some point, I decided that when I was eighteen, I'd try it just because I could. By the time I turned eighteen, however, I'd decided I hated the smell of cigarettes and had four younger siblings watching. I skipped it. I've never been very motivated to try things just because they were forbidden, but I know others who are the opposite. It's likely a temperament or personality thing.

The forbidden fruit effect specifically refers to *never* being allowed to have something. If we look at this through the lens of reactance theory, reactance comes into play only if a child knows about the food they have never been allowed to eat *and* they felt that not having access to that food reduced their freedom, which doesn't seem as common of a scenario. Usually, a child eventually tries the food in question. Let's say you don't allow your child to drink soda, but they see other kids at a party drinking it. If they truly never try the soda *and* they have adopted the idea that they are really missing out without it (forbidden fruit effect), then reactance could come into play. But in my experience, a child will get curious and try it even if they're not "supposed to," or they will get served it accidentally because another parent doesn't know they aren't allowed. In that case, the forbidden fruit effect could no longer apply.

There's no body of research on the effects of delaying the introduction of hyperpalatable foods to kids as a form of restriction. It could be an incorrect application of the forbidden fruit effect, similar to what has been said about alcohol. Some people entertain the idea that delaying alcohol consumption in modern kids makes them drink more later, but researchers have observed that kids who have been delayed from alcohol exposure longer tend to have lower alcohol consumption and risk of alcohol misuse later (although the observational research does not determine whether delaying alcohol was the cause of less alcohol misuse). There's a difference between not being allowed to eat something that you've never tried, and not being allowed to eat something you've tried and loved. No one knows what will happen to your child if you take this approach, but as with everything, it's likely a combination of how you approach it, your child's temperament, genetics, modeling, and numerous other factors.

QUESTION #6

"If my child is eating too many cookies away from home and I'm not there to stop them, how can I get them to choose more moderate portions on their own?"

The goal of embodied independence is to help kids get in touch with, respect, and take care of their bodies, which also means, for most children, not eating large amounts of hyperpalatable foods. We work hard to give our kids a balanced environment so that, as they get older, eat away from the family, and start to have more agency, they will eat in their best interest. Yet too often, that's not what happens. Kids get hyped about candy at a birthday party and they may eat a lot of it even if they have a stomachache. One mom told me her seven-year-old daughter's friends were giving her daughter "junk food" at school and then the daughter wasn't hungry to eat the nutrient-dense lunch she brought from home. The family already spoke positively about all types of food at home, served some hyperpalatable foods, and her daughter knew what different foods did in her body (including the foods in her lunch from home). The mom wanted to know what she should do to have her child refuse the snacks from her friends. Some kids are going to pick up embodied independence, absorb what a balanced diet is, and learn all about food quickly. Other kids will have a harder time based on their temperament or brain chemistry. They may be highly affected by hyperpalatable foods, and if that is the case, it's unreasonable to think they will make the decision to pass on the "junk food."

It can be tempting to immediately jump to sharing negative information about hyperpalatable foods to try to convince your child to avoid them, but there is another option that I believe is less likely to cause worry, guilt, or shame related to eating, while still protecting your child's nutrition. Keep building up your child's embodied independence at home and deliberately alter what you're offering at home. If your child is eating cookies at school, you might consider not serving cookies on school nights at home. If your child is eating hyperpalatable snacks with friends, you could avoid those foods entirely at home. You can also include your child by giving them a choice so that they know what to expect—"You can have cookies at school or at home tomorrow. Which would you like?" (Only do this if you believe the conversation would be positive for them.) Then decide whether to serve cookies based on whether they ate cookies at school or not. Leaning into the principles you will learn over the next few chapters can help balance what is happening when your child is making their own decisions.

INTUITIVE EATING

Intuitive eating is a term that frequently comes up when I'm discussing restriction with parents. I might ask, "How many cookies are your kids allowed to eat?" and a parent might respond, "Oh, we don't restrict them," citing intuitive eating as the model they adhere to. However, there is some confusion out there surrounding intuitive eating, which I'd like to clear up here. Intuitive eating is a therapeutic approach that was originally created by two private practice eating disorder therapists, for adult women who wanted to move past disordered eating and regain the embodied independence they had lost in their experience of diet culture. These two therapists wrote a book called *Intuitive Eating*, and the approach became quite popular.

As we look to understand the research on intuitive eating, it's important to understand that research surveys that measure it aren't measuring how well people are following the framework in the book *Intuitive Eating*. They are studying the four following concepts:

1. **Unconditional permission to eat**—There are no rules or diet plans that dictate what, when, or how much an individual eats; there are no forbidden foods; the individual eats whatever they desire to eat in the moment.
2. **Eating for physical rather than emotional reasons**—An individual copes with negative feelings without using food to manage emotions, stress, or boredom.
3. **Reliance on hunger and satiety cues**—The individual trusts their body to tell them what, when, and how much to eat, and when to stop eating.

4. **Body-food choice congruence**—The individual desires to nourish their body with nutritious foods that will help them perform well and give them energy and stamina.

Recently, it has been suggested that the intuitive eating approach should be used to prevent the development of disordered eating in children. Some researchers have begun using this framework with tweens and teens as part of eating disorder prevention programs, where participants learn to reject weight-loss-diet mentality, increase their interoception, understand the dangers of strict food rules, and respect their bodies' need for movement and nutrition. Thus far, based on a very small number of studies, these programs show promise. As a first step toward determining how intuitive eating might affect younger children, researchers have begun to study parents. Parents who use an intuitive eating approach have been observed to have a more permissive feeding style and keep more fruits and veggies and less salty food and soft drinks in their homes. They tend to think their weight is "just about right" and have higher economic status. However, there is no evidence yet of the effects on younger children.

The four elements of intuitive eating largely align with those of embodied independence—at least for adults (and in some cases adolescents) on a therapeutic eating journey. For example, these elements help people meet the body's nutrient needs; rely on hunger and fullness cues; and discourage the characterization of foods as "bad" or "good." *Unconditional permission to eat* is another one that can help individuals become more embodied by improving interoception or relieving the reactance that some weight-related diets produce. The hope is that it will eliminate an adult's desire to overeat foods that were taken away as part of a diet and instead turn inward to respond to their body's internal signals.

Here's an example of what this might look like for an adult. The other day, I opened a small bag of potato chips. I happen to know that if I eat the whole bag of this brand (as I've done many times), I will end up feeling nauseated. I also know that if these potato chips are in front of me while I'm working, I will slowly finish the bag, even after I'm satisfied, even if I'm feeling nauseated. I enjoy potato chips frequently, and I attach no morality to potato chips. To use intuitive eating language, you could say I give myself "unconditional permission" to eat potato chips. I am in no way physically or emotionally deprived of potato chips, yet the hyperpalatability gets my brain every time. If I'm paying close attention to what I'm eating and how I feel (rather than working while eating), however, I can tell when I'm satisfied and I will put the bag away. Or if I know I'll be working while eating, I might pour some chips out next to the rest of my lunch and put the rest of the bag away. That day, I intended to work through lunch (not ideal, but real life), so I poured out some chips and put the rest of the bag away. That's the effort it takes me, an adult, to resist the food industry's attempts to get me to purchase and eat larger amounts of hyperpalatable foods than I want to, while also enjoying potato chips. This is the only way I can have unconditional permission to eat, while also honoring my satiety cues and my desire to leave room to fill up on foods that won't make me feel queasy.

It would be asking too much of a child, however, to eat with this level of mindfulness, especially with hyperpalatable snacks. I can understand why parents who have used intuitive eating methodology and practitioners who exclusively guide adults through intuitive eating might assume the same methods could *prevent* disordered eating in children, perhaps by improving their sense of embodiment. However, there is minimal (in fact, none, to my knowledge) evidence to back up the efficacy of this approach to prevent disordered eating in children, and it neglects a holistic approach to embodiment, which is embodied *independence*. Some parents may have a child who is minimally affected by hyperpalatability or they may be able to carefully craft their home food environment and routines in such a way that they can teach independence while also letting their child use all of the intuitive eating strategies. But this is the exception. As parents, we can't expect children to be able to navigate the current food environment on their own when it's designed to hijack their embodiment. They need our support and guidance to learn how.

GIVING YOUR CHILD STRUCTURED PERMISSION

To restrict or not to restrict? When parents ask me about this, I recommend an approach that I call *structured permission*, which looks a bit different for every family, but that always involves a combination of clear boundaries and attentiveness to your child and their needs. If restricting hyperpalatable foods risks being too controlling, and unconditional permission to eat risks asking too much of a child, then structured permission is a middle ground that allows us to create healthy boundaries around food that also nurture embodied independence. But instead of thinking in terms of restriction—which can feel limiting and strict—structured permission invites us to think about the other side of the same coin while also motivating children to be fully embodied.

With structured permission, the *how* of implementing these boundaries may be especially important. A couple groups of researchers have observed that restricted kids are more likely to have higher diet quality when their parents also have high warmth and responsiveness with a moderate level of boundaries. There may also be fewer conflicts with boundaries when different parents have the same ones and consistently hold them. Being warm and attentive to your child's needs in such a way that they feel connected to you is an essential component of being able to say, "Everyone gets two cookies today, and we'll have more with lunch tomorrow." Holding food limits with warmth reinforces your connection with your child. Structured permission also means practicing patience, listening to your child, providing snuggles, and staying calm or using humor to redirect behavior in tense situations. It also means avoiding language that could make a child feel shamed for eating or wanting to eat something.

Recently, a first-grade teacher shared the following story about one of her students with me. This child, a picky eater, was struggling to find something to eat for lunch in the school cafeteria. "My mom said I can't eat any more bread this week," she told her teacher. This school always offers sunflower seed butter and jelly sandwiches for kids who don't like the main offering, but the little girl seemed unsure of what to choose because she didn't like what was being served and she wasn't allowed to eat any more bread that week. I share this story as a counterexample of what warmth and structured permission look like. This type of restriction likely stems from a parent's disordered mentality surrounding food and could indicate internalized weight bias and body dissatisfaction on the parent's part, which can be passed down to the child.

Structured permission, by contrast, sets boundaries in a way that supports a child's embodied independence. These boundaries might include:

- Not bringing large amounts of hyperpalatable foods into the house
- Creating consistent yet flexible routines related to foods
- Serving "child-size" portions of certain foods
- Considering your child's perspective when creating routines related to accessing favorite foods
- Providing access to limited amounts of hyperpalatable foods

Alternatively, boundaries that could more easily lead to a more controlling or harsh form of restriction could include:

- Basing food decisions, including portions, only on a parent's perspective
- Requiring obedience to food rules with no exceptions
- Using guilt or shame to control a child's food intake

- Providing no access or no consistent access to hyperpalatable food so a child doesn't know when they will have access
- Routinely hiding food

The way we model eating food and feeding affects how our kids respond to their bodies. So if our goal is to help our kids be embodied and live healthful lifestyles, we must look inward first. If we have unchecked disordered eating, weight stigma, or internalized weight bias ourselves, the "structure," "boundaries," or "limits" that come naturally may in fact be controlling forms of restriction that unintentionally extend that disordered eating into our homes. So the first step in developing structured permission is prioritizing ourselves. A mom recently told me she was in eating disorder recovery and was afraid she would pass her eating disorder on to her kids. I reminded her that prioritizing *her* own recovery is likely the most important thing she can do to improve *her children's* relationship with food. We're often told to "put on our oxygen mask first," which can feel like another item to add to the endless to-do list of life. This is different. I'm not suggesting you add yourself to your to-do list. I'm suggesting you choose the type of structured permission you will use based on what will support *your* relationship with food and your body as well as the development of your child's embodied independence.

WHAT DOES STRUCTURED PERMISSION LOOK LIKE?

If you have decided that structured permission is the right approach for your family, you may be wondering what that looks like, practically speaking. I recommend following these steps:

STEP 1: DELAYED INTRODUCTION

Start by delaying introduction of hyperpalatable foods (or whatever food you are specifically focused on restricting). If your child is a baby, put off the introduction of hyperpalatable foods until at least age two, if possible. If your child is a toddler and there are hyperpalatable foods they have not yet tried, you can choose to delay them. Let's say you are eating a slice of pizza, and your child doesn't yet know what pizza is—you can choose to give them something else. A child cannot feel they have lost the freedom of eating a food if they haven't yet been exposed to or tried the food. And if they do vaguely know about it, but have never tasted it, there's still an opportunity to delay before it becomes a "thing" for them. Once they've had the food and know it's something that could be part of their life, you can move into the next phase—strategic exposure.

STEP 2: STRATEGIC EXPOSURE

If there are foods you can't delay—or can't delay anymore—it's time for strategic exposure. Strategic exposure involves allowing your child to feel satisfied and unrestricted, even as you're reducing their access to hyperpalatable foods. It's part of nourishing your child's embodied independence and making it more difficult for hyperpalatable foods to hijack their developing brain.

Strategic exposure might look like taking a limited quantity of a snack out of the bag and putting it on a plate, or serving food in a smaller bowl or cup (five jelly beans in a soup bowl looks empty and sad; five jelly beans in a tiny dip container looks full and cute). Other examples of strategic exposure include:

- Making a food item smaller so they get more (four small cookies might be the same as one big cookie)
- Serving a small amount of the food more frequently
- Diluting juice with water
- Not buying the hyperpalatable foods your child hasn't asked for
- Not eating restricted foods in front of your child

We recently implemented strategic exposure in our house by getting some new, kid-friendly dishes. We're a big ice cream family, so we incorporated optional nightly ice cream into our bedtime snack routine. This worked for us, except the kids' self-serve portions were getting bigger and bigger, to the point where my husband and I knew our current strategy wasn't serving them well. So we bought some cute little inexpensive ice cream sundae dishes. They hold about a scoop of ice cream (a lot less than the soup bowls they had been using). The kids complained about getting less ice cream a few times, but within a few weeks, they were used to the new dishes and content with how much ice cream they had. In our case, the kids knew that we'd changed the size of the dish to decrease portion sizes, but often with strategic exposure, kids don't realize they are being limited—and they still feel they are getting everything they need and want.

It's important to point out that some elements of strategic exposure can also be used as part of weight-loss-diet culture. I don't like that, but it's the reality. So, if just reading about those strategic behaviors fosters a diet culture mentality for you, then they probably aren't a good fit. And even if they *are* a good fit, these strategies don't need to be rigid. They aren't rules, and it isn't a failure if you try these and they don't work for you or your child.

For some parents, the goal of structured permission might just be to implement some boundaries, whether they are around increasing the intake of certain foods or decreasing others. If this sounds appealing to you but you don't know where to start, try beginning with one simple boundary that will support your child's nutrition needs and go from there. Some examples I've seen parents use with sweets (but that can be used with all hyperpalatable foods) include:

- No more than one sweet a day
- Certain nights of the week are dessert nights (the child chooses which nights to have dessert)
- No processed sweets, but homemade treats are okay

Boundaries like these can be implemented clearly, warmly, without drama, and in a way that supports your child's embodied independence.

STEP 3: COLLABORATION

If your child is old enough, you could consider including them in some of your decisions around structured permission. In my house, it is easier to enforce limits that our kids have had some input in establishing. They push back against them less. Researchers in other areas of child health have observed the same thing: Collaboration can reduce reactance.

As an example, for many years, our kids were allowed to eat an unlimited amount of candy on Halloween. As they got older and stayed out longer, however, the large amount of chocolate (and hype) on Halloween night made going to sleep difficult, and we found that they were grumpy and sleep-deprived throughout the week after Halloween. So one year, we decided to set a limit on how many pieces of candy they would each eat on Halloween. We brought it up with them like this, "Hey, for Halloween this year, how many pieces of candy do you think would be good to eat?" One kid suggested five pieces. The other one wasn't particularly interested in the conversation and said, "A thousand." We went with five pieces, and that was that. There wasn't any drama.

In another phase of life, the kids weren't getting much nutrition in their bedtime snacks, and given the whole picture of their diet, we decided that bedtime snacks needed to change. Rather than telling them they weren't allowed to have certain foods at bedtime, or that they were making bad choices and demonizing the foods they were choosing, we told them they could choose from a list of bedtime snacks we provided that filled in some of their nutrition gaps. There were lots of options on that list of foods they are willing to eat, and they got to choose. While we were setting the structured permission, we were also inviting their collaboration by giving them choice.

No matter what your version of structured permission looks

like, make sure you're paying attention to how your child reacts and implementing your limits in a warm and non-shaming way. If your child is always crying because they only get one cookie, maybe that's a sign that one cookie is not satisfying enough. If they are showing signs of shame related to eating, maybe they need less structure and more access to all foods. It's okay to experiment. What matters most is the *how*: how you're delivering your message to your child and whether they feel they are being listened to.

SPEAK INTENTIONALLY

When it comes to structured permission, your words, tone, and body language matter. They communicate your beliefs to your child. To start, don't say more than you have to. When you talk about what your child is or is not allowed to eat, avoid adding on "qualifications" like "You can have a piece of cake, *but only one, because it has a lot of calories / is bad for you*," as opposed to, "You can have a piece of cake." Adding qualifications is a place where negative comments about body and shaming can easily sneak in. Our qualifications, tone, and body language must be positive, or we lose the opportunity for structured permission and are left with only restriction.

In general, whether you are setting a limit or holding a boundary, I suggest sticking to the basics, while also validating that it's normal and just fine to want more. You might say something like "There are no more cookies available for this meal. I know, they are the best chocolate chip cookies, and I want to eat more, too. We'll have more tomorrow!" Or, "I know you want to have candy for breakfast. It's tough to wait until after lunch." If your child gets upset, don't try to reason with them or explain why you have a limit in that moment (for older kids, it might be helpful to tell them you will explain why later in the day when everyone has cooled down). Just empathize. It's hard not to get what you want. Help them calm down as much as they are able to, and move on with the day. Learning to be okay with disappointment is important. Embracing discomfort is a part of life, and it's a key element of eating with embodied independence, for parents *and* for kids, which we'll talk more about later in this chapter.

TAKING THE PRESSURE OFF

While I encourage you to do your best at sticking to your menu and eating routine, teaching your child to eat with embodied independence usually means letting them determine how much they will eat. One common way parents override their child's sense of embodiment is by pressuring them to eat more. By "pressure to eat," I mean forcing your kid to finish all the food on their plate if they say they're full, or making them eat if they say they aren't hungry. It's normal to want to make sure our kids eat enough or not too much, especially if we're concerned about them being underweight or picky. It comes from a good place, because we want to make sure our kids get what they need to thrive! But researchers studying pressure have observed that pressuring kids to eat is associated with struggles that include increased child anxiety, picky eating in childhood, unpleasant mealtimes, eating because of the sight or sound of food instead of hunger, more emotional eating, disordered eating symptoms, and less enjoyment of food. A common misconception is that pressure contributes to unexpected weight gain, but this is not supported with research at this time. People may have also heard that pressure to eat definitively decreases a child's ability to eat intuitively, but there is very little research on this, and it has mixed results, with some showing decreases in intuitive eating and others showing increases.

If you often find yourself pressuring your child to eat, or if you're generally experiencing stress around your child's eating, I recommend making "no pressure" your new normal. If your child says they are full after three bites, go with it. If they say they aren't hungry at all, go with it. If food waste is a top concern for you, as it is for many parents, try to serve smaller portions when you aren't sure how much your child will eat. This has the dual benefit of helping them tune in to see if they are hungry, which builds their interoceptive skills, and reducing waste.

It's important to point out that pressure is not always associated with negative effects and we don't know how much parents pressure their kids because of their child's eating struggles or how much the pressure from the parents causes the negative effects. Many studies have observed no connection between pressure and the quality of a child's diet, or a negative association for some of the kids in a study and a positive association for the other kids. Pressuring a child doesn't guarantee your child will be affected in a negative way—and if they *are* affected, it's unlikely they would experience all the negative outcomes associated with pressure to eat.

We have a perfect opportunity here to use the practice of curiosity, as well as common sense. Consider your own child—who they are, their temperament, their physical health, and whether they seem to have trouble with interoception. For example, some kids don't like to be pressured, and if you tell them what to do, they will dig their heels in. That's just their personality. Other kids get anxious when they are pressured and it makes them lose their appetite. In other situations, pressure may be an important part of keeping a child healthy by requiring them to eat a certain amount because their interoception is currently impaired in some way. If that's the case, then *how* you pressure and whether you can use it to help with embodiment rather than simply overriding it will likely make all the difference.

EMBRACING DISCOMFORT

A few years ago, my son had a rough soccer game. He didn't play his best, and his team lost in a landslide. He was really upset. I wanted my little guy to feel better, and as we walked to the parking lot, I saw an ice cream truck and thought, *I could get him some ice cream, and that will make him feel better.* But then I thought, *I don't usually buy ice cream from ice cream trucks, and he hasn't even asked for it. I would only be doing this to make him feel better so he wouldn't need to be sad, and I wouldn't have to be uncomfortable with him being sad.* Basically, giving him ice cream in this specific instance would be feeding him for emotional reasons.

In the end, I didn't make the offer. Instead, I did something very uncomfortable for me. As we got in the car, I said, "That was a hard game." We were sad together the whole way home, and I listened to all the unhappy things he had to say. Then we moved on with the day. It wasn't fun, and there weren't any heartwarming moments during that car ride. But in the end, I felt like both of us got a little bit more experience sitting with negative emotions instead of trying to make them immediately go away—a skill that's not my strong suit and something I need to develop. I hope the experience will help me the next time something hard happens. Life is full of discomfort, and we need skills to manage that discomfort without completely avoiding it or letting it flatten us.

An interesting thing happened after the sad soccer game. I shared the story on social media. I made it clear that I don't always choose the path of discomfort—other times, I might have purchased the ice cream, I'm not judging anyone who would have bought ice cream, and eating ice cream to handle emotions isn't a moral failing. Most people appreciated the point I was trying to make—that always trying to make our kids' discomfort go away isn't going to build their capacity—but a small group had a different take. They thought not buying the ice cream was an example of diet culture and fatphobia, something that would perpetuate disordered eating. Which is worth considering. Could my decision not to "fix" this sad moment with food erode my child's embodied independence and contribute to disordered eating?

THE IMPORTANCE OF DISCOMFORT

Discomfort wasn't a topic on my radar until a few years ago. Articles about discomfort generally don't pop up in child feeding and nutrition research or education. I was introduced to it from a different angle, when I found myself avoiding some business-related tasks because they made me anxious. The avoidance was starting to cause me more problems, to the point that I found myself poking around the self-help side of the internet until I came across the phrase *avoidance coping*. I bought some books on the topic and quickly learned that, in my daily life, I am likely a little too comfortable.

For some people, modern conveniences have translated to a very comfortable life. If I don't like a show or a song, I have millions of others to choose from. I can learn the definition of a word or get the answer to basic questions in a matter of seconds. There's a large amount of instant gratification. Plus, I have endless ways to distract myself from anything uncomfortable, including those pesky business tasks. So when things go wrong or get at all messy, I don't have the same skills to deal with it that someone a century ago would have had. I need to deliberately build up my capability to take it in stride and do what needs to be done. My discomfort with discomfort doesn't do me any favors, since life in general is full of discomfort. I need to be able to handle it.

As I was learning some skills to get myself back on track with my business tasks, it occurred to me just how relevant the issue of discomfort is to many elements of feeding kids. Discomfort pops up when we have to put in the effort of cooking or obtaining nutritious meals, when we have to deal with whiny and grumpy kids when they're hungry, when our kids are upset and we know they can be soothed with foods, when our kids aren't eating in the way we hoped they would, when family meals go awry, and more. We have a never-ending supply of opportunities to feed kids for the primary purpose of removing their (or our) discomfort. This is helpful when that discomfort is actual hunger, or when they feel full and we let them stop eating. But it can be unhelpful if feeding is the go-to for helping kids calm down or to keep them busy.

SITTING IN YOUR DISCOMFORT

Plenty of people lean toward eating when they feel upset or bored. No judgment. As I've mentioned, I've been known to stress-eat potato chips myself! Researchers have observed that some kids are more likely than others to eat for emotional reasons. We don't know exactly why, but there are many correlated factors, including temperament, genetics, sleep, and kids' ability to cope with emotions and negative thoughts. It may also be related to parent modeling and how they cope with their own emotions, as well as whether they manage their child's emotions with food. As in other areas of child feeding, parents and kids likely influence each other. For example, if a child soothes easily with food, the parent will figure that out and use food to soothe the child as needed.

I have no moral quandaries with using food as a pick-me-up. At the same time, it's not healthy for us if that's the *primary* way we handle negative emotions. When we eat for the purpose of handling feelings, we're often not embodied, and it may work against our physical health. We may be out of touch with our hunger, fullness, or the feeling that's telling us what our bodies really need in that moment, and we may eat foods that crowd out the foods that meet our nutrient needs. We also may be denying the consequences of avoiding our emotions.

Why is it so important to learn to tolerate uncomfortable feelings? Well, at the most basic level, these are feelings that are going to come up throughout a person's life, so learning to cope in a healthy way is a tool that will have a long-term payoff. But when it comes to food specifically, difficulty coping with negative feelings has a relationship with disordered eating. Using food for emotional regulation can be a risk factor for disordered eating and is also a symptom of some clinical eating disorders. Additionally, children with higher stress levels have been observed to be more likely to have disordered eating. Researchers have observed that children who avoid confronting their sources of stress have a higher likelihood of disordered eating than children who have the same level of stress but don't avoid their problems.

To be clear, teaching your kids to tolerate hard emotions without using food is not the same as giving them a hard time for eating in difficult moments. I am not suggesting that you guilt or shame your child for choosing to eat ice cream to feel better after they placed last in a race. This is *not* fostering their embodied independence, and it's potentially worsening their relationship with food or enforcing weight stigma. You can take a more embodied approach by saying something like, "Ugh, I bet that coming in last in that race was really hard." Then give them space to talk and listen to what they have to say. An embodied approach may even involve food: "That was a really hard loss. Let's go spend some time together. We can go to the playground and then get a snack afterward," or "We always go out for dinner on race nights. Where do you want to go tonight?"

Sometimes feeding kids for reasons other than hunger is more about quelling our own discomfort than our child's. Toddler and preschooler tantrums can be intense. Big-kid outbursts and the things they say can be brutal. Parenting all day or after a day at work, sibling fights—it's all hard! Facing tween boredom makes weekends long. Whether it's the noise level of the shouting or the bloody nose from a toddler headbutt, being around our amazing kids is sometimes overwhelming and very uncomfortable. Who wouldn't use food if it worked quickly to diffuse some of the tension?

This isn't about *never* using food to take the edge off. Sometimes it really is the right tool for the situation. But it's important to cultivate our other tools as well. The tools that help me include breathing exercises, remembering that it's not my job to keep my child happy all the time, learning to talk more about my emotions and helping my kids learn to talk about theirs, and making sure the kids have activities to do beyond just snacking when we're traveling. These practices have all helped me to tolerate uncomfortable feelings so that I don't rely on food or snacks to always do the work for me.

The truth is, sometimes the practices of feeding aren't fun. It's uncomfortable to tell your toddler (or tween) that ice cream isn't on the menu. It's uncomfortable to listen to your child have a tantrum when you know a snack would fix it immediately. It's uncomfortable to watch your child eat two bites of dinner. It's even uncomfortable to see your kid feel the sensation of hunger, even if they aren't starving and food is coming soon. Hangry and "starving" are different from "a bit hungry." Preventing a child from responding to their hunger cues under the guise of "practicing discomfort" or "not eating emotionally" (when what the parent is really concerned about is their body shape or size) is well within the bounds of diet culture and even disordered eating. And it's important to remind ourselves that we're working on helping our kids build embodied independence, and that includes experiencing moments of reasonable discomfort. This book is about building confidence, and it's only in difficult moments that we can use and grow our confidence.

These situations are often nuanced, so it's essential to practice curiosity when you are contemplating whether to serve food during a tough moment. It can help to ask yourself four critical questions:

- *My child is asking for food, but are they actually hungry?* If the answer is no, then it's an opportunity to consider all the options available to help them with their emotions.
- *Am I giving my child food to escape my own feelings, such as frustration, annoyance, or guilt? And are my feelings caused by their boredom, sadness, or other emotions?* If the answer is yes, it's an opportunity to reflect on all the options available to you in this moment to work through your own emotions.

- *Am I approaching this situation from a diet culture mentality that is focused on body shape and size or rigid eating rules?* If the answer is yes, it's an opportunity to reflect on your weight bias and what options are available in this moment that will strengthen your child's embodied independence.
- *If I offer food in this moment, will I be challenging my child's physical health by crowding out nutrients that they need, or making it more difficult for them to listen to their hunger and fullness cues?* If the answer is yes, it's an opportunity to think about the range of foods that could be offered at this time, as well as alternatives.

The reason to ask yourself these questions is so that you can have greater awareness of why you are doing what you are doing when you are using food for comfort. It's not to cause shame. I might use these questions and realize I am planning to use food to soothe my child's and my own discomfort, *and* it may negatively impact their nutrition for the day. And I might make the conscious decision to serve food anyway, because my other child was up sick every two hours last night, and I'm in survival mode. In that moment, I can eschew guilt and I can *also* choose to plan for tomorrow so that I'm a bit more conscious about the kids' nutrition and meal timing, to help things balance out over the course of a few days. I might also push myself to not use food during a tough moment later in the week, to build up our family's discomfort skills. Awareness can sometimes reveal an urgent need to change our actions. A parent may see that their rigid approach to feeding is coming from a place of weight bias and dieting mentality, or a manifestation of disordered eating in themselves or their child. In that case, they may want to push themselves to embrace a new approach to eating and feeding as quickly as they can, perhaps also seeking guidance from a health professional.

It can be very difficult to abruptly stop using food as emotional support. If someone doesn't have tools to use instead of food, they may have emotional outbursts toward themselves or someone else, turn to other substances or addictive habits to replace the food, or become depressed or anxious. They may end up in a worse position than if they had kept eating snacks. If you or your child hasn't yet discovered other tools for coping with stressful situations, don't start by eliminating food from those moments. Instead, start with learning more about emotional regulation strategies, talk to a friend who has been through something similar, or get in touch with a person qualified to provide emotional, mental, or spiritual guidance. Then start to use those strategies instead of food.

REMEMBER: FOOD CAN BE LOVE, CARE, AND COMFORT

After I had each of my kids, some friends set up a "meal train." Friends and neighbors brought us dinner a few days a week for several weeks. Well over a decade later, I still remember many of those meals and what people said and did. I still feel grateful and cared for. During a rather overwhelming time, these meals were a show of emotional support that decreased my discomfort.

During a recent Thanksgiving holiday, as we do most years, we celebrated with my husband's family. In general, his family enjoys slightly different foods from what my family does for holidays (we're more canned cranberry sauce and pumpkin pie; they're more homemade cranberry sauce and apple pie). I appreciate the different traditions and usually don't have much of a drive to make a pumpkin pie myself. This year, though, I missed the tradition of my family's favorite foods enough to get cooking. I made a bunch of dishes and sliced the canned cranberry sauce. I was full by pie time, but I didn't hesitate to enjoy my slice, because it had an emotional purpose. It brought back memories, and every bite was delicious.

I left the table stuffed and happy. The next day, I brought back another tradition by eating pumpkin pie for breakfast.

One of my kids: "Are you eating *pie* for breakfast?"
Me: "And eggs. Want some pie?"
Kid: "No."
Other kid: "I don't like pumpkin pie."

Their loss—I got all the pumpkin pie.

Meals can feed our souls, bring comfort, soothe our pain, support us through hard times, play a practical role in making us feel good when we feel bad, and so much more. That's all good stuff. Let's make sure that we don't lose the forest for the trees when it comes to embracing discomfort.

There's nothing fun about the practice of embracing discomfort. However, it's an essential piece of the puzzle. When we combine curiosity with a willingness to embrace discomfort, while continuing to practice embodied independence in the way we eat, it helps us make the changes we decide are right for our families. It enables us to keep going even when we don't have all the answers, or when change feels hard. And that might be the case more often than not.

Nurturing embodied independence isn't easy. It requires a lot of us as parents—looking out for and reducing exposure to the thin ideal, encouraging and developing interoception, establishing our "restaurant," resisting the temptation to pressure our kids, and being willing to sit with discomfort. Often parents focus on only one element of this practice. They may choose to focus on teaching their child to stop eating when they are full, but in the name of promoting a positive relationship with their body, they may allow their child to snack throughout the day on whatever they want. I also see parents who are nailing balanced meals at routine times but are openly discussing how these meals can contribute to weight loss—their own or their child's. Eating with embodied independence means looking at the bigger picture, as best as we can. We don't need to do all these things perfectly—no one can. But in a combination that works for our families' needs, these practices can help us help our kids listen to, trust, and care for their bodies.

3

EAT TOGETHER

"If we move dinner up to 5:00 PM, when am I going to work?" my husband asked. It was 2020, and we were splitting our days between childcare and our paid jobs. I would work in the morning, and he would work in the afternoon and evening. We had recently come to the realization that with the stress of the pandemic, our kids needed an earlier bedtime, and to make that work, they needed to eat dinner earlier. If we all wanted to eat dinner *together*, we would also have to juggle our work schedules. In this case, that meant we would both end up working after the kids went to bed, which is what we did.

It wasn't the first time we'd had this conversation. Family meals (dinners, specifically) are one of our core family priorities. As soon as my husband and I became parents, we took advantage of our flexible schedules to make family dinners possible. We juggled and planned, turned down opportunities or invitations when necessary, cut back on work achievements, and avoided most activities that took place at dinnertime. When my first son was born, we would put his infant chair in the middle of the table while we ate so that he could be part of the experience. When my second son came along, we would pull his swing up to the table so that he could join the fun, too. We've gone through many rough patches with kids not wanting to sit or come to the table. We've had messes, sibling fighting, and times when no one had the capacity to cook.

But through it all, we've held fast to these family dinners. Prioritizing them has meant that even when it feels like we're trying to move mountains to eat together, we keep doing it and we make it work as best as we can. Why would we do this to ourselves?

On one hand, my husband and I both grew up in homes where our families ate dinner together. Eating together feels like tradition, and it feels important to us. Beyond that, however, there are hundreds of research papers about family meals, and most researchers conclude that family meals can be a powerful force for good, associated with mental and physical health benefits, and opportunities to implement other parenting practices, like curiosity and nurturing embodied independence. If the trick to navigating the ever-present food noise is to make choices based on the needs of the specific people in your specific family, then family meals are an ideal place to get to know your family's eating tendencies. They are something worth prioritizing.

I define the term *family meal* as any meal or snack where a child eats with at least one adult. I like this definition because it acknowledges that meaningful connections can happen in different ways. One spring, my son's baseball team held practice and games during dinnertime. Because the season was important to my son and changing dinnertime wasn't our best option, we embraced a different style of family meals for those few months. We had two dinner shifts, one parent and one kid at each. It turned out to be great. It was one-on-one time, connecting over food. Sometimes my husband or I need to work or to be somewhere else during dinner, so at those family dinners, the other parent gets the kids to themselves. It's always a different vibe and offers a new way to connect.

In your home, family meals might mean that only kids are eating together—without an adult. This may not offer parental modeling, but these meals have their own social benefits. I've seen kids eat foods they wouldn't try in front of adults because all the kids at "the kids' table" were eating them. Peer pressure can be a force for good.

Many years ago, my mom shared one part of her approach to

family meals, and I love it so much I want you to hear it, too. She always had seventy-five irons in the fire—like many moms do—cooking, caregiving, juggling jobs, homeschooling, and doing all the things. As my siblings and I got older, often someone was missing dinner because of work or activities and came home to eat after everyone else was long done. This is what she told me that she chose to do: "I decided that no one needs to eat alone. When someone sits down to eat, I stop whatever I'm doing and sit down with them." It's not the same as a family meal where everyone is eating, but even the act of sitting together captures some of the magic. It's connecting, and that's powerful. Rather than getting caught up in whether you're doing family meals exactly right (there's no such thing), focus on the connection and the food.

Of course, not everyone is going to be able to—or want to—move mountains to make family meals work. My husband and I had some time flexibility over the years thanks to a combination of being in school, having jobs that allowed working from home sometimes or flexibility with hours, or being self-employed. We often also had short commutes, and consistent schedules since our jobs did not have changing shifts. Plus, there are two of us. All of which is to say that we had the option to move mountains, while other families don't. So while I won't shy away from saying that family meals can have a big positive impact on a child's health, I want to acknowledge that family meals may not be realistic as a "best" practice for everyone. If family meals don't work for your crew right now, that's okay. Give yourself a break, feel free to skip this pillar, and move on to the next one.

BETTER CONNECTION, BETTER HEALTH

When my older son was three years old, we were a few months into telling knock-knock jokes at dinner. Suddenly, my younger one, who wasn't yet two, said, "Knock, knock." We all looked at him, surprised, and said, "Who's there?" He smirked and said in his adorable toddler voice, "Banana face!" We were all delighted together.

Family meals are about more than food. They are opportunities for us to spend time with our kids and connect. Eating at the same time in the same place brings us together in a unique way. It allows us to share the details of our days, ask each other questions, escape the constant pinging of app notifications or the distractions of screens, and hopefully have a laugh. During meals, we can teach our kids social skills or to be considerate of other people, and we can share more about our values. In today's overscheduled world, adults often have jobs or other obligations that demand a lot of time and energy, while kids have school and might be in various extracurricular activities. Days pass quickly, often with almost no chance to slow down and talk about the things on our minds. Family meals can be anchoring moments where we tend to our physical and mental health.

Plenty of tangible benefits have been tied to family meals. Researchers have observed that children in families that eat together are more likely to have lower levels of anxiety, depression, and suicidal ideation. And the benefits aren't just for children. Parents who hold family meals tend to have better mental health, higher levels of family functioning, more self-esteem, lower depressive symptoms, and less stress. It's reasonable to wonder whether parents with better mental health are simply more likely to plan family meals, and I'm sure that is true. Still, some researchers observed a decrease in depressive symptoms among parents who served family meals, even after removing those who were experiencing depressive symptoms before the study. This suggests that family meals may have mental health benefits all on their own. Plus, dinner is a time when our kids can bring up something tough that happened earlier in the day, which gives us a chance to support them. Without that consistent scheduled time together, we wouldn't have as many of those settled moments that lend themselves to conversation and connection.

Carving out time to eat with your kids is also an excellent opportunity to lead by example. Modeling can be very powerful. It isn't the only factor that affects what kids eat, but when children see their parents or other trusted adults eating a variety of healthy foods on a regular basis, they will be more likely to try what they see the adults eating. I'd venture to guess there's also motivation for parents to serve a more balanced meal when the entire family is eating together. That's certainly the case in my house. I'm more likely to cook a full meal when we're eating as a family because I want my kids to have the chance to eat all the things they need to meet their nutrient needs. Not to mention that I want to eat something that tastes good to me.

Researchers have observed that children who eat family meals do in fact eat higher-quality meals and have a higher-quality diet. And it starts young! Even though meals with little ones can absolutely be stressful (*see:* the tantrums, mess, and distractions), some researchers have observed that infants and toddlers in families that eat together enjoy eating food more. Kids who have family meals have also been observed to eat more fruits and vegetables, and fewer salty snacks (although that's not always the case). This is also true of parents—parents who have frequent family meals tend to eat more fruits and vegetables. For some children, family meals are associated with less picky eating, and researchers have observed that kids who have more frequent family meals have less disordered eating, eating disorders, and better body satisfaction. These are mostly observational studies, so we can't say that family meals *cause* these outcomes, but still, the association is there. It's commonly stated as fact that children who have more family meals engage in less risky behaviors, such as violence, early sex, drug use, and alcohol use, and that they do better in school, but the research on this is mixed.

One of the most rewarding benefits of family meals, as I see it, is often overlooked. They create a space for the entire family to practice gratitude and learn about food justice. Every person should have access to enough food and variety that they can meet their nutrition needs. If we're sitting around a meal, we have food. What a gift. Whether it's simple or fancy, cooked from scratch or heated out of a box, the food is there. And mealtime can often provide an opportunity to model gratitude together through a moment of pause, a song, or a prayer, and to have conversations about food.

Talk to your children about where their food came from. A farmer grew those tomatoes. A migrant worker picked them. You bought them and prepared them. We can also talk about the injustices of how little farmers and workers are valued and paid, and ways we might be able to help by supporting local farmers. If we never have to go hungry or cut back to make the food stretch, we can talk about how lucky we are. We can talk about the problem of hunger, why people don't have enough food, and ways that we can help through food drives or working at a soup kitchen. If we're fortunate enough to have a variety of nourishing food choices available to us, we can practice being grateful for that. We can talk about the injustices of food deserts, places where people don't have access to a variety of foods, and we can wonder what it would be like to never have our favorite foods available to us. We can talk about the fact that some people don't have the choice to eat a variety of foods for many different reasons—from lack of access to disabilities to poverty—which helps dispel the myth of sole personal responsibility for health.

These conversations about food justice will likely be infrequent, and they should never be used to try to guilt or shame your child into eating. Telling a child to "finish your dinner; there are starving children out there!" is completely unhelpful. Instead, we can look for opportunities to share information naturally and factually, because if we have enough to eat, we can't forget those who don't.

MAKING THE MOST OF EATING TOGETHER

While you can make family meals whatever you want them to be, there are some goals to keep in mind to maximize the benefits. These aren't hard-and-fast rules, because as with all the practices in this book, what your family meals look like will be determined by who is in your family and what they need. Still, these guidelines can be helpful as you begin to envision what you want family meals to look like in your home.

In terms of frequency, the more meals your family can eat together, the better. Researchers have observed greater mental health and nutritional benefits the more meals that a family is able to eat together, with the "magic number" being seven meals or more per week. It doesn't matter which meals you eat together, and even snacks can be quick family eating opportunities. If you can't hit seven meals a week together, don't let that discourage you. You can still strive to eat together whenever it's possible. Each family meal is valuable. My son and I went to a coffee shop one day when he had a half day at school. He ordered hot chocolate, and I bought a two-pack of peanut butter cups. We shared the peanut butter cups and decided they taste better when we eat them together. Ever since, we always share our two-packs of peanut butter cups. If you're not eating together at all, start with one meal or snack a week. Every little bit counts.

One of the goals of eating together is nurturing embodiment, so aim to limit screens at family mealtime. Screens distract us and make it harder for us to hear hunger and fullness cues, they interrupt our connection with one another around the table, and they make it difficult for children to get the food exposures (seeing, smelling, tasting, etc.) they need to learn to eat new foods or move beyond picky eating. In fact, researchers have observed that when the TV is on during family meals, often there are no longer benefits associated with the meals.

For some parents, putting kids in front of a show at lunch, for example, is the only way they can get a moment to themselves. Other families declare Sunday night football-and-pizza night and eat in front of the game. That's all fine! Every meal that your family eats together doesn't have to fit the "ideal." This isn't about being rigid; it's about establishing a ritual of eating together and using that time to connect in your household.

Finally, remember to find the fun amid the chaos of cooking, spilled food, and complaints. Fun can go a long way toward helping everyone be relaxed and connect in a positive way. Adding playfulness, games, and silly conversations to mealtime—whether that's by telling jokes, playing twenty questions, or singing into your broccoli like a microphone (my husband's personal favorite!)—can really lighten the mood.

If fun feels impossible because there's a lot of fighting, negative body talk, pressure to eat, or tension, the family meal structure we're talking about in this chapter may not be the best choice for your family right now. My family has had our fair share of upsetting mealtimes, or phases when there seemed to be more spills and drama than eating. For all the recommendations that family meals can have benefits, it's important to note that there are circumstances in which family meals can do more harm than good. For example, if a family is not functioning well overall, or if there is a lot of talk about weight or weight-related teasing, pressure to eat, or negative experiences during the family meals, researchers have observed that the children present at these meals are more likely to develop disordered eating.

When my own family has had a harder time with family meals, my husband and I have had to stop and think about what was going on and how we could adjust to make dinnertime positive again. We've changed the time that we all sit down together, we've told stories as a short-term distraction, we've eaten dinner while watching a movie, and we've considered taking a break from eating together (and we've been glad when sports have mixed up the dinner routine). As I mentioned earlier, if family meals are not working for your family for whatever reason, skip them. Let each kid eat when it's convenient for them, or prepare separate meals for each child if that's what needs to be done. Wait until you're in a different life phase to reconsider.

EATING NORMS AT THE FAMILY MEAL

One night, when my sons were two and four, I was feeding them solo and I wanted to use up some salad before it went bad. I didn't think they would want the salad, so I just put it all in a serving bowl for myself and gave them different foods for their dinner. I got through one bite of my salad before one of the kids said, "Hey, why is that all yours?!" He had recently learned that you shouldn't eat out of the serving bowl, because you're supposed to share with everyone. "Oh, I didn't think you would want any," I said. After being left out like that, both kids wanted a whole plate of salad, and I barely got my fair share.

What you eat as the parent is an important part of family meals. In some studies, researchers observed that children ate more nutritious meals during family meals, but only if the parent was also eating more nutritious meals. There are benefits to your child's eating when you all eat the same meal. Your enjoyment of nutritious foods can be contagious in the best way. Of course, there are many situations, like when someone has a severe allergy, that make it impractical or unhelpful to have all family members have the same meal. But you can still model eating a variety of foods, even if you're eating slightly different foods from your child.

If you have a picky eater, you would probably find yourself doing a little dance of celebration if your child ate your share of the salad (I did). One common strategy that parents of picky eaters often use to increase food variety is a *one-bite rule*, in which a child is required to at least try a bite of all foods that are served as part of a meal. Tasting can be a great way for kids to learn to like new foods and have a more varied diet. For some kids, the one-bite rule can be a tool in helping them learn to try to enjoy foods they typically wouldn't touch.

At least one experimental study concluded that tasting foods (for both neurotypical and neurodivergent children) reduced children's anxiety. If a one-bite rule is encouraged and implemented in a positive way, it can be a tool that builds a child's embodied independence, even if tasting new foods is uncomfortable for them. You can help your child tune in to their body by using warm, positive language like, "Let's try this new food together!" or "This salad is crunchy to me. What does it feel like for you?" As long as you are taking the opportunity to connect with your child during the meal, allowing them to stop eating when they're full, and not using shame or punishment to get them to eat, you are helping your child develop their sense of embodied independence with the one-bite rule. At the same time, it is possible for the one-bite rule to become a stressful and even traumatic practice for some children if they feel high levels of pressure to try foods that are uncomfortable to them. The one-bite rule may cause feelings of not being in control of their body, especially if they experience shaming or anger from whoever is enforcing the rule. If this is the case, the one-bite rule is working against a child's embodiment as well as the connection with their family. If you're using this rule and it's causing tears or refusal, or it's making one person sit at the table for a long time after everyone else is done or is leading to punishments, then it's probably not working. It's making eating and mealtimes a negative experience. In your family meal experiment, the results are showing you that the one-bite strategy is not a good fit.

My family hasn't used a one-bite rule. It likely wouldn't have been a good fit for our temperament mix, although my husband and I worked at helping the kids learn to try new foods. At the same time, when I introduced the idea to one of my sons when he was about six that his body needed to taste something eight times before it knew if he liked it, it flipped a switch for him. Suddenly, he was willing to push past some discomfort to get his eight tastes in. And it quickly expanded the number of foods he would eat. (I haven't been able to find the research reference for this "eight tastes fact" again after initially reading it, so I can't call it *factual*, but it certainly worked for him!)

One caveat to the one-bite rule: Don't call it a "no thank you" bite or "one polite" bite. It's one thing to have a rule that "we always try a bite of the foods on the table at home." It's another to suggest that your child is impolite or ungrateful unless they try a food or that they can't say "no thank you" in certain circumstances. As kids go out and to other people's homes, being able to say no to a food that they are allergic to, that doesn't align with their values, or that makes them feel sick is an essential skill. Also, forgo using food as a reward for trying a bite. In other words, don't say, "You can only have dessert if you take a bite of this carrot." For all the disagreement in the research on other topics in child feeding, researchers consistently observed that rewarding with food either doesn't have an association at all (meaning it doesn't do anything) or is associated with the things we generally don't want, like more eating in the absence of hunger, food conflicts with parents, or eating fewer "healthy" foods and more hyperpalatable foods. If you really want to reward your child for trying new foods, consider praise and nonfood rewards, as those have been observed to encourage eating variety. By using nonfood rewards for a short time to help get a kid over the difficulty of trying something new, you can then wean them off the reward system as they build their own desire to eat the foods.

Family meals are a great opportunity to offer "adventurous" foods to your child, since you are there to support them, discuss the foods, and create a positive environment. Still, as I've mentioned, be sure you also serve a familiar food that your child will reliably eat, especially if your child has severe picky eating issues. This does not necessarily have to be a favorite food or a hyperpalatable food. A familiar food is any food that your child is comfortable with and usually eats—even if it's "boring." In fact, sometimes pairing boring familiar foods with foods a child hasn't yet learned to like makes the unliked foods a bit more attractive. Your child may be more likely to try the stew if it's served with boring rice on the side than if it's served with their favorite mac and cheese. When there is a food that your child is comfortable with, even if it's boring, you can be confident in standing your ground that you will not get up and make another meal.

I'm often asked whether you should let your child eat as much as they want of their preferred or familiar food. What you choose to do is completely a matter of personal preference, philosophy, and culture. If you would like to take an "all foods are equal" approach, then let your child eat as much as they want of any food, including the preferred food (this may be especially relevant if a parent is addressing their own disordered eating or for an extreme picky eater). If you want to focus on expanding tastes and getting kids to eat their meal, you might let a child eat a serving of their preferred food and require a bite of everything else before having more of the preferred food (this may be especially relevant in the case of having a mild to moderate picky eater or a distracted kid). If you find that your child will eat *only* their preferred food if it's there, without being willing to try the other foods, you may choose to offer only a limited amount of the preferred food (also relevant in cases of mild to moderate picky eating or poor interoception). And if you want to make sure certain nutritional needs are being met, or if your goal is to reduce food waste, you might require that if a child is still hungry after eating their preferred food, they need to first fill up on the foods already on their plate, and if they are still hungry, they can ask for more of their preferred food (this may also be relevant if a child has some forms of disordered eating, or is a distracted kid).

Speaking of food waste, one common concern when parents are introducing new foods is how much of any food to serve. There are "official" portion sizes from various public health sources, but I find these are really useful only in cases such as government nutrition program requirements (schools must give children one serving of juice, which is four ounces), nutrition facts labels (there is 40 mg of calcium in a half cup of this food), or nutrition recommendations (this person needs to eat four servings of cooked greens per week, which is two cups). When it comes to your child, the right portion size is what your child will eat. Instead of thinking in terms of portion sizes, I think in terms of *starting portions*—how much you put on your child's plate that they'll be willing to eat.

If you're requiring your child to try a food they don't like yet, consider serving a *micro-portion*, or a very small taste, like one pea or half of a spoonful of soup. You already know they probably won't eat more, so that one taste will keep you from wasting food. For their preferred food, on the other hand, serve a full portion. In general, try your best to be thoughtful and realistic. I find that parents often serve wishful portions, heaping on the plate however much they think their child "should" eat to be healthy. Often, this is more than your child will want. Having too much on the plate can influence a child's eating, causing them to eat either more or less than they would normally. Err on the side of smaller portions when you are unsure—it allows children to listen to whether they are still hungry. Once you have a better idea of your child's appetite, likes, or dislikes, you might make the starting portions bigger or smaller.

Family meals, and all the variables that go with them, will change over time, especially as kids grow into teenagers. Maybe your child is on the school basketball team and practice runs late, or they're always trying to eat and run because of their homework load. Maybe your child's starting portion sizes need to change, or you decide to try implementing an "explorer bite" for your picky eater. Adjusting to family circumstances is what feeding your kids is all about. When you consider the potential mental and physical health benefits that come with family meals, it's worth evaluating your mealtime environment and how you find a doable way to eat together. It might be challenging to press through a rough patch, reorganize your schedule, and find fresh ideas for playful dinnertime conversations, but when you embrace eating together as a valued ritual in your family and experience the connection that hopefully comes with it, you may find it was completely worth it.

4

EAT WITHOUT JUDGMENT

When my son was four years old, he came home from preschool with a question: "Is chocolate bad?"

I asked him why he was wondering. He said he'd heard it from a classmate.

"Some foods do a lot of things in your body," I responded. "Some foods do a few. Chocolate does a few. But there are no bad foods."

"Oh, okay," he said and moved on with his day.

The story doesn't end there, however.

Two years later, at six years old, he came back from school and said, "My friend says chocolate is unhealthy, but some foods just do a few things in your body, right?"

"That's right," I said. "If you only ate chocolate, you would be unhealthy, but what would happen if you only ate broccoli?"

"You would be unhealthy."

"Right."

Turns out, chocolate is a controversial food among kids. Two years later, when he was eight, my son said, "My friend said chocolate is unhealthy. I told him that chocolate just does a few things in the body, but he didn't get it. But he also wouldn't get it if I asked him what would happen if he only ate broccoli. He would think he would be healthy, but he wouldn't!"

I mostly listened and empathized. He was right, and he was

willing to stick up for the facts that he knew. He had the information he needed.

During our most recent conversation about chocolate, my son was ten, and the conversation shifted. This time, he talked about how everyone he knows says that chocolate is bad or unhealthy. I could sense that the easy days of "what my parents say is right" were coming to an end. Because when "everyone" says one thing, and "Mom and Dad" are the only people saying another thing, Mom and Dad may need to back up their claim. Now my son is starting to wonder a lot more about *why* his friends say chocolate is bad.

As parents, it is our job to talk with our kids about all aspects of life, from seat belts to teeth-brushing to friend troubles. And we spend a lot of time talking about food. One research group looked at the conversations a group of moms were having with their kids and observed that 15 percent of those discussions centered on food! We talk about what we'll eat for the next meal, what our kids may want from the grocery store, which snacks to pack for an after-school activity. Given how often food comes up in conversation, we need to think critically about the impact of what we say and how we say it. On a deeper level, this is about the way that our attitudes and judgments related to food affect our kids' ability to eat with embodied independence. This brings us to the fourth pillar: Eat without judgment. A key piece of raising kids to eat with embodied independence is about countering the two loudly blaring food messages that they will be exposed to constantly in the world beyond your kitchen:

1. Food is bad or good, healthy or unhealthy; and
2. You should eat a lot of hyperpalatable food

MESSAGE #1: "FOOD IS GOOD OR BAD, HEALTHY OR UNHEALTHY"

> "In my class, one of the preschoolers told another preschooler that his mom put poison in his lunch. It ruined the relationship between the two families."

> "In school, my son was told that pizza is unhealthy. He has ARFID and now he won't eat pizza, which had been one of the few foods he was willing to eat at school."

> "Learning that her body needs colorful, healthy foods has helped my daughter overcome her picky eating."

These quotes are just a sampling of the thoughts parents have shared with me related to the messaging their kids hear about foods. One prominent mainstream message of our time is that foods neatly fit into categories of "bad" or "good," "healthy" or "unhealthy." The bad, unhealthy foods are the ones with a lot of calories, saturated fat, sugar, salt, additives, processing, pesticides, heavy metals, and other toxins. The "good" and "healthy" foods are the ones that are low in calories, processing, and toxins and high in things like antioxidants, fiber, protein, specific fats, phytochemicals, and probiotics. We all know in general which foods tend to be called *healthy* or *unhealthy*. We see these messages often, and so do kids. Information about nutrition and health is plastered on packaged food items and blasted by all forms of media. It's shared by other kids on playgrounds as well as by adults around them.

Even comments that seem positive—like the "colorful, healthy foods" one above—showcase how information about food might change a child's thoughts or actions related to that food. People categorize everything. It's how our brains work. Children's brains, starting as young as two years old, will begin to sort information into food categories, whether we are consciously teaching them these categories or not. They will learn that there are breakfast foods and dinner foods, foods that only go in bowls, foods that are only appropriate for certain occasions, and so on. They'll learn about food groups and how foods are prepared. Kids will also internalize the healthy and unhealthy food categories—they're nearly impossible to avoid—and start to sort foods this way, too. However, if we want our children to have the freedom to eat without judgment, we need to offer alternative frameworks for thinking about food.

There are many reasons why foods have come to be thought of as morally good or bad, or simply healthy or unhealthy. The thin ideal and weight bias is a big part of it. For many people, food is an integral part of cultural identity, and in various religions, certain foods may be allowed or forbidden, moral or immoral. Food can also be used as an indicator of an individual's social class. Generally, more privileged groups shape the societal discourse about which foods are healthy or unhealthy, with "clean whole foods" being viewed as morally superior in our current era, as opposed to "ultra-processed foods." Based on current research, certain eating patterns have been associated with poor health and chronic disease, while others have been associated with good health. Many of us implicitly think we are on moral high ground when we eat "good" foods and that we are doing something wrong when we eat "bad" foods. Researchers have observed that people hold this belief whether they have a disordered relationship with food or not.

From a practical standpoint, categorizing certain foods as *healthy* or *unhealthy* is an unhelpful simplification. If a person with diabetes is having a low blood sugar episode, soda could save their life. If a child has an allergy to salmon, this "superfood" could be life-threatening. To say foods are *good* or *bad* is confusing, especially because a lot of people disagree about exactly which foods are healthy and which foods are unhealthy. Most adults I meet have some skepticism about nutrition information because they see headlines all the time talking about how certain foods are good for you, but then a few years later, public opinion flips and the foods are considered bad. Margarine is an excellent example. For a while, it had the spotlight as the better alternative to butter, until we learned the partially hydrogenated oils in it were damaging to our health (they were banned in 2018). And kids seem to be confused, too—parents have told me that their children ask why their teacher told them the muffin in their lunch was "unhealthy" when it was made of lentils and oats, for example. Additionally, inconsistencies from parents—saying something like "Candy is bad for you" but then also "If you clean your room, you can have candy"—can result in conflict with their child over "healthy" and "unhealthy" foods.

In the eight years that I have been answering nutrition and child feeding questions from the public, I am constantly asked a variation of the same question: "Is it healthy for my child to eat ____?" Parents have asked about bread, green veggies, beans, grains, meat, fish, rice, fruit, potatoes, tomatoes, candy, frozen foods, eggs, and virtually every other food or group of foods you can think of. The fixation on foods being simply good or bad is adding a significant amount of stress to parents' plates.

When parents hear negative information about food, they also may think of that food more negatively, be less likely to purchase it, and remove it from their child's diet. This may be fine if the food is something like boxed macaroni and cheese, because the nutrients in that meal are found in countless other foods. It's damaging, though, when it comes to avoiding things like fruits and vegetables (because of fear of pesticides), or other protein-rich foods, which are not as easily replaced. Variety is where we get our "nutrition insurance," because different foods give us different nutrients. It's also where we get our protection from harmful things in foods. I like to say, "Every food has a downside," because in a sense, it's true. There are contaminants, heavy metals, or harmful chemicals in all foods. This is true of every food. When we eat a variety of foods, though, we are less likely to get too much of one kind of contaminant. And while it's fine to remove some foods from your diet, remember: We all have to eat. Sometimes when I'm feeling especially snarky, I remind people that the fastest way to become unhealthy from food is to not eat it at all.

Perhaps you think this argument is ignoring just how dangerous some of the "bad" sides of food really are. After all, there are entire books, social media accounts, documentaries, and speakers dedicated to sharing just how extremely "healthy" or "unhealthy" certain foods can be. However, the next time you see a post or article that vilifies a particular food, approach it with a critical eye, remembering that creators get more attention and engagement from viewers when their messages are more extreme. These extreme messages also create fear, which is good for selling products. It's not that selling products or wanting attention is bad (if you're a creator, that's your job). But keep in mind that people may present information in a particular way to try to get you to do something that will benefit them perhaps more than it will benefit you.

If influencers and headlines are two big sources of good/bad food messages, kids also have another source of these extreme messages: their parents. Someone recently told me they tell their kids sweets are "death snacks" and that processed foods are "garbage." I'm guessing that might ring some alarm bells for their child. I've heard kids pass judgment on all sorts of foods. A few years ago, an eight-year-old told me in a judgy tone, "I thought school lunches were unhealthy." This child was from a family rich in food resources and nutritional knowledge, which allowed his parents to have choices about what to eat and to take specific approaches to food. But every day, he was taking this perspective to school with him and possibly stigmatizing his classmates who were getting school lunch, which is not at all uncommon.

Your kids may come home from school with comments about who ate what, or what eating style their friends have (vegetarian, kosher, gluten-free, etc.). Food stigma is real, and it has a real effect on children. In fact, researchers have observed that children with access to free school lunch often don't eat those lunches due to the stigma.

There is also a long history of racism baked into the categorization of foods as "healthy" or "unhealthy." A classic example: If you say kale is healthy, no one bats an eye, but if you say collards are healthy, everyone says, "Well, it depends on how they are cooked."

Even though both kale and collard greens are "healthy" in the same ways, and both can be found with bacon pairings, collards are often called out as potentially unhealthy in the media and nutrition circles. Racism plays a big role in the stigmatization of foods common in the Black population of the Southern US, such as collards, fried chicken, sweet potato pie, and biscuits.

THE IMPORTANCE OF FLEXIBLE THINKING

Our practice of categorizing foods as "healthy" or "unhealthy" is worth questioning. Does all the information help our kids make "better choices," contributing to their independence? Or does it cause disordered eating, hurting their embodiment? There isn't much research on children in this area. However, researchers have observed that adults with disordered eating tend to have a more rigid "good versus bad" perspective on food. Researchers have also hypothesized that rather than outside information *causing* someone to become a rigid thinker, some people already think rigidly, so they find it easy to implement a two-category system of food.

Does the binary categorization of foods as "healthy" or "unhealthy" decrease the likelihood of a child developing disordered eating, or does it contribute to disordered eating? Even when we pull together research related to eating disorder prevention and nutrition education, we don't get good answers from the research, so the short answer is: "We don't know, but it probably depends on the child." If a child is very embodied and doesn't have much internalized weight bias, learning some foods are "unhealthy" and eating them less, or learning some foods are "healthy" and eating them more is a good thing for their embodied independence. If a child, however, has a tendency toward disordered thinking about food and their body, then this could fuel disordered eating or an eating disorder. In the face of such unclear research, it's a good opportunity for curiosity and common sense. Yes, our kids need information to nurture their independence, and also, we should be aware some types of information might make disordered eating worse in some children.

Beyond "healthy" versus "unhealthy," it's also worth noting that categorizing food as "toxic" versus "clean" can be a symptom of disordered eating. *Orthorexia*, or *orthorexia nervosa*, is a term that is becoming increasingly popular to describe disordered eating where the main feature is a person obsessively eating only "healthy" or "clean" foods—to the point of damaging their physical or mental health, or social relationships. This is not an official eating disorder diagnosis on its own, but it does overlap with some other diagnoses. As of early 2026, there is no consensus on the definition of orthorexia in the research or healthcare fields, but healthcare providers agree that the effects of this way of thinking can be very dangerous to people's health.

If a child is at risk for developing an eating disorder (due to factors like family history, temperament, perfectionism, or internalization of the thin ideal), it can only help to encourage flexibility in their thinking about food and to reduce their exposure to binary healthy/unhealthy thinking. Of course, you cannot completely shield your child from healthy/unhealthy messaging, but you *can* model a different way of thinking and talking about food for them that will help build their flexible-thinking muscle. You can use the scripts in this chapter and avoid using good/bad language about food at home. If your child has risk factors or a special interest in considering whether foods are good or bad, I urge you to consider a more neutral approach to food with your child. Avoid justifying your use of good/bad language by claiming it's healthier to have a "clean" diet than to have a healthy relationship with food. A child can have a healthy lifestyle without such a black-and-white mentality about food, and if disordered eating ever develops, you will already have been practicing a more flexible mindset around food. If you find yourself struggling to give up a two-category food model, it might be an invitation to consider whether inflexible thinking may be informing your own attitudes about food.

Even if you think you've "said all the wrong things" because until now you've talked about foods only as healthy/unhealthy, it's never too late to change your strategy. If your child is young, you can simply change the way you're speaking. If your child is older, you can make this an opportunity to model changing your mind. What a powerful skill to be able to show your child. You might say something like this:

"I've been thinking about how I used to call certain foods 'healthy' and other foods 'unhealthy.' I've changed my mind on that. Lots of foods can be healthy or unhealthy depending on how we eat them. I'm going to practice calling foods by their names and seeing how I feel when I eat different foods. I might learn more about what foods do in my body, too. Let me know if you hear me calling a whole group of foods healthy or unhealthy."

MESSAGE #2: "EAT A LOT OF HYPERPALATABLE FOODS"

Food companies' number one goal is to hook us as lifelong consumers of their products by creating positive emotional associations between us and their products or brand, starting when we are children. When I was growing up, my great-grandma often gave us parmesan fish-shaped crackers and pretty cookies that came out of fancy white bags with a picture of a farmhouse on them and a top that folded down. To this day, I cannot see that logo or bag style without fondly remembering how delightful it was to be spoiled by my great-grandma. So of course I still buy their products. This is especially true for companies marketing hyperpalatable snacks and drinks like fast food, chips, and soda, with the messaging that we'll be happier if we consume their product. Even if your child is too young to ask for a specific food, they've been seeing bright colors, logos, and smiling faces on packages from their infancy, and eventually, they'll request a snack or dessert or cereal from the specific brand with marketing that appeals to them.

Food companies try to create this positive relationship in similar ways that the tobacco industry historically did in Black and

Hispanic communities to instill widespread use of their products. They may sponsor community events, Little League teams, local school needs, park projects, and scholarships to gain community trust and buy-in, while also putting up their signs, making their products readily available in the community, and targeting the community with advertising to children. And the similarity is not a coincidence: Many tobacco companies acquired hyperpalatable food companies in the 1980s, so they had a marketing playbook ready to pull from.

Despite the happy messaging that surrounds hyperpalatable foods, the reality is that eating too much of them can lead to poor health more easily than eating "normal palatable foods," because hyperpalatable foods fill us up without delivering the nutrients we need, among other issues. A hyperpalatable food like ice cream doesn't have to be categorically "bad" or "unhealthy" for us to acknowledge that it's unhealthy to eat ice cream for every meal, and that if we did, we would not be getting enough protein or magnesium. Many kids *are* eating too many hyperpalatable foods, which are in turn crowding out the foods that would otherwise meet their nutritional needs, keep their blood pressure stable and their cholesterol down, and support their mental health.

Food companies conduct extensive research into how to override hunger and fullness cues to engineer foods that people will consume in high volume. Many children are still learning to recognize their internal cues, or else they simply cannot recognize these cues due to the way their brains are wired and thus are especially vulnerable to the draw of hyperpalatable foods. Even adults are susceptible. Earlier, I gave the example of how I've found myself eating too much of the brand of chips that I like because it tastes so good that I don't recognize I am full until I am *really uncomfortably* full. I've learned to listen to my body better, but it takes time.

It's not just the food engineering. Advertising has also been shown to make kids eat more than they would have otherwise, as well as to affect the brain region associated with rewards, driving children to make food decisions based on enjoyment rather than how full or satisfied they are. If kids aren't taught about food marketing, they may get the impression that they're somehow "bad" if they are eating "too much" of a certain food. But once they're old enough to understand concepts like deception or manipulation, it's fair and reasonable to explain to kids that food companies try to override their hunger and fullness cues to get them to eat more and buy more food.

I found myself trying to explain this to my son during a recent trip to the store, when I had to tell him that no, "fruit snacks" were not fruit, even though the package had the phrase *real fruit* all over the box. Fruit snacks are candy, I explained. He would feel very different eating an apple versus a package of fruit snack "apples." Fruit snacks are fun, and they aren't "bad," but the deception used to market them *is* definitely bad. Similar advertising ploys are used for a wide variety of foods, including those that claim to be "Made with real cheese!" (a very tiny amount of "real cheese" amid everything else) or "Contains vegetables!" (a tiny amount of vegetable powder) on the packaging. Food pouches for babies and toddlers are also notorious for saying they contain kale, pumpkin, or other vegetables, when they are almost entirely applesauce.

It's not just that the advertising and marketing of hyperpalatable foods is ubiquitous—hyperpalatable foods themselves are everywhere. In schools, at the pool, the corner store, the hotel, the gas station. Some communities have fast-food restaurants on every block. Constant exposure to these foods (and their advertising) makes a person hungry, and if they are what's immediately available and affordable, they're what a person is going to eat.

DELIVERING YOUR OWN MESSAGES

Your child will undoubtedly be exposed to good food / bad food messaging and hype around hyperpalatable foods. That doesn't mean they can't also be exposed to different messages, too. You can offer up your own messages—ones that will help them develop a positive relationship with food and with their body.

It's important to note: There's no perfect way to speak to a child about food. There's not even a "best" way. There are just ideas for *how* to do it. I have a few favorite messages that I use to give kids a helpful framework for thinking about food as they interact with the rest of the world. You may choose to use some of these phrases with your kids, or you may come up with some of your own. But these messages go much further than telling kids that foods are either healthy or unhealthy.

"What I eat doesn't make me good or bad."

Years ago, as I waited in the office to register my son for school, I watched the principal stop and grab two chocolate candies from the candy dish on her way to her office. As she did so, she said, "I'm so bad!" Personally, I thought it was smart to bring a moment of enjoyment to her day given the number of disgruntled adults and students she regularly had to interact with!

I think most of us want to be able to eat without guilt or worry. We want our kids to have a *morally neutral* approach to eating so that they can be free to enjoy food, life, and their bodies. Whether your child is a picky eater, an adventurous eater, has a massive sweet tooth, or anything else, food itself is morally neutral, and what your child eats doesn't make them a bad or a good person. Recognizing this is one of the hallmarks of eating with embodied independence.

When we're talking directly with our kids about foods, or talking where they can overhear us, we can trade out some of the language that suggests that we're good or bad people based on what we choose to eat.

Instead of saying: "I'm so bad for eating chocolate."
Try saying: "I love chocolate. I'm going to enjoy this!"

Instead of saying: "I was good today and ate all my veggies."
Try saying: "I feel good from all those veggies I ate today."

Instead of saying: "I worked out and earned my dessert."
Try saying: "I'm so hungry after working out. Dessert is going to taste so good."

We can do this even if we're talking about wanting to eat differently in the future because something we've eaten doesn't make us feel great now.

Instead of saying: "I was so bad and went back for thirds. Now I'm stuffed and my stomach hurts."
Try saying: "Whew, I'm stuffed! That was delicious. I feel like I need to take a nap."

Instead of saying: "I shouldn't have eaten all those potato chips because I was feeling sad. Now I'm feeling so nauseated."
Try saying: ⟦silence⟧

Declaring that you are "good" or "bad" for eating certain foods is not the same as following a certain diet that is part of your ethical, religious, or moral beliefs. In these cases, food may have a moral value based on your beliefs about what one should or should not eat, or how a food is prepared or how an animal is killed. Following your religious and ethical beliefs is important, and I'm not suggesting you stop doing that. Within the boundaries of what foods are allowable for you, though, there are often still "healthy" and "unhealthy" foods that don't need to have any morality tied to them. Those allowable foods can be morally neutral. For example, I'm not aware of any moral or ethical code that prohibits all added sugars all the time.

All that said, declaring foods morally neutral is not the same as saying, "All foods are the same, and it doesn't matter what we eat." All food can be morally neutral, *and also* every food is going to do something different in your body. Additionally, all food can be morally neutral, *and also* we can choose to eat different amounts of foods or eat them in different ways based on how they make us feel in our bodies. Food is not all the same, which is why it's important to recognize that while we are gradually teaching kids that foods aren't intrinsically bad or good, we can also teach them that different foods do different things in their bodies. It's two sides of the same coin.

"Every food does an important job in my body, and my body needs them all."

When my son was in preschool, I was asked to come in and talk to his class about why we eat fruits and vegetables. I didn't want to go in and just say foods were healthy or unhealthy. That didn't seem like useful information for children, and I wanted to offer them some useful information. Some parents feel strongly that when it comes to kids, the less food information they have, the better. They believe kids will have a better relationship with food if it's not "complicated" by information. While I appreciate the motivation behind this idea, and I can understand why someone might believe it, given how much food information kids are exposed to outside of the home (whether we like it or not), it's just not realistic. Raising a child without exposure to nutritional information would require a sheltered upbringing with a carefully controlled food environment in the home. This might be possible for a few kids, for a few years, but it's not a common experience. When talking to my son's class, I wanted to give the kids a reason to eat certain foods that made sense to them. So I brought in a laundry basket full of a rainbow of fruit and vegetables and told them:

> Red foods help your heart.
> Orange foods help you see in the dark.
> Yellow foods help your cuts heal.
> Green foods help you fight off sickness.
> Blue and purple foods help you have a strong brain.
> White foods give you energy.

The reason we benefit from eating fruits and vegetables truly is because they are different colors, and each color (or the chemicals that create the color pigments) does something different in our bodies, which I explain in more detail in the next chapter.

"I can listen to my body to find out how to eat best for me."

My son played in a doubleheader soccer game where someone provided a snack in between games. The snack was hash browns from a fast-food restaurant. Not all the kids ate them—my son didn't, because they were from a restaurant he doesn't like—but I noticed that the ones who did visibly "wilted" and did not play well during the second game. My son and I had a conversation after the game. We talked about the difference between how the kids who had the snack felt after eating it versus the kids who hadn't. I told him that they would have played better if they had eaten that snack *after* the game. We talked about how it's okay for us to have fun foods like fast-food hash browns, and we also can think about how they will affect us. They don't help us with playing soccer well, so we might pick a different time to eat them.

The next week, a parent brought some sweet grain bars that gave the kids quick energy for the second game, and the kids perked up and played well after eating them. I pointed out that difference to my son as well. Both the sweet grain bar and the hash browns were fun foods, both were morally neutral hyperpalatable foods, both okay to eat, but they had different effects on the body. That information can help him decide what he wants to eat for soccer performance between games in the future *and* assure him that fun foods are okay, too.

Sometimes when I notice different feelings in my body because of eating different foods, I try to share that with my kids. I might say something like, "Now that I've eaten, I don't feel angry anymore," "That hot chocolate made me feel warm and cozy," or "I'm so sleepy because I ate so much cheese. I have to go take a nap." (Now they even remind me, "You're going to need a nap if you eat that cheese, Mom.")

Listening to our bodies might also mean considering information gathered from blood work or doctor's exams and responding to what our bodies need based on that information. This may lead your family to remove certain foods from the home or to serve some more than others, but this is part of kids learning that food is an important part of their health.

"Food companies are tricky and are trying to get my money."

Research suggests that if we want adolescents to be able to resist food marketing, they need to be able to recognize food marketing when they see it, they need to understand the effects of food marketing and how to defend against them, and they need to have the cognitive ability and motivation to resist the marketing. That's a tall order even for teenagers, and we wouldn't expect kids under fourteen to be able to do it at all. With this in mind, the number one way to decrease the effects of food advertising is to reduce your child's exposure to it. This is significant enough that Canada's national food guide explicitly recommends limiting kids' exposure to food marketing. Limiting kids' exposure to food marketing is easier said than done, and it will likely take extra effort. But it might include avoiding commercial TV and streaming services that show commercials, muting the radio or podcasts when commercials come on, taking food out of packaging before serving it, or buying generic-brand foods. And these aren't the only strategies to use.

Another way to potentially lessen the effects of food marketing is by encouraging negative emotions in your child about the marketing as well as the companies executing it. With a younger child, you might use language like, "That commercial is being tricky and trying to get us to do something like buy their snack." Educating a child that something is food marketing alone doesn't change the outcome of the marketing—they will likely still want the food or have positive feelings toward the brand. But you *might* be able to slightly weaken the effect of the marketing by disrupting some of the positive feelings the companies are trying to instill in your child.

As your child gets older, you can begin to teach them more about the motivations of food companies, how their practices may harm people and communities, and how to recognize when a food company's actions don't align with your family's values. One marketing technique that food companies commonly use to target teens is to position "junk food" as a form of rebellion and freedom. Research shows that this marketing technique works by exploiting the developmental stage when a teen wants to establish their identity outside of their parents. Another study showed that by appealing to middle school–aged children's (especially boys') sense of injustice at the damage hyperpalatable food marketing was causing to their community's health, they were able to decrease the children's positive association with food companies and their products. Many of these children decided to drink less soda and eat less "unhealthy" food. Instead of rebelling against parents, they were rebelling against the manipulation of food companies.

If you decide to teach your child about food companies and their marketing strategies, make sure you are directing the negative feelings toward the food company, not the food itself! You might say something like, "Food companies are trying to get us to pay extra for a sports drink by telling us you'll be a superstar player if you drink it. That's not true. Is this still something we want to buy?" In my house, the answer is "sometimes." We buy sports drinks for certain situations, like during long sports games, but we don't buy them when we don't need them. We don't let the companies trick us into giving them our money when our bodies don't need sports drinks.

"Don't yuck on my yum."

Whether it's keeping your comments to yourself when your child covers their pasta with ketchup or teaching your child not to say negative things about someone else's food, it's just good practice to avoid commenting on what another person is eating, unless it's something positive like "That looks good!" We don't need to judge what our family, friends, or classmates are eating. The more positively we speak about foods, even if they aren't foods that your child is willing to eat yet, the more you open possibilities for them to try new foods and appreciate people who eat differently from how you do. This is important for respecting other people's cultures or backgrounds as well as people they will interact with.

NUTRITION INFORMATION AND FOOD SCRIPTS BY AGE

It can be a great learning experience to share nutritional information with kids, and it can help their relationship with food. However, in certain scenarios, it can also stress kids out and have the opposite effect. Again, we need to think about *how* we are delivering this information. We don't need to be talking about nutrition facts constantly. You can bring up the topic of nutrition now and then, just like you would anything else. But don't overdo it—there is such a thing as too much of a good thing.

Sometimes kids give us the opportunity to offer information by asking questions. When one of my sons was eight, we were eating some purple cabbage as a family with lunch, and he asked, "What does this food do in your body?" Magic words. The next thing everyone knew, they were getting a lesson on how antioxidants get rid of free radicals in the body (I'll just own the fact that I'm a nerd). Sometimes an interesting nutrition fact comes to us while we're shopping or cooking or eating. "Hey, guys, did you know carrots help you see in the dark?" That's a fun way to share something.

If you find yourself sitting at the dinner table intensely telling your child that they need to eat all the carrots on their plate because the vitamin A helps them see in the dark and they will lose their night vision if they become vitamin A deficient . . . well, you can imagine how unpleasant that might make the meal. It could easily lead to a power struggle and encourage them to push back against eating any of their carrots at all. In some cases, this dynamic could lead you to pressure them to eat more food altogether, potentially challenging their sense of embodiment. Try putting yourself in your child's shoes at mealtime. Most of us don't want to talk constantly about the health benefits of our food—we just want to enjoy it! Also, remember the practice of curiosity. If your child doesn't express curiosity about nutrition information, don't push long conversations on them. If your child is interested, tell them more.

When teaching your child about nutrition, there are six guidelines to keep in mind:

- Use the correct names of all foods.
- Share interesting facts about how the food affects the body in ways that are meaningful to a kid's life.
- Teach that foods are morally neutral and that different foods affect our bodies differently by sharing facts as opposed to opinions or judgments.
- Provide engaging experiences with foods, including teaching your kids how to grow, prepare and cook, or taste them.
- Allow the facts and information you share to become more complicated over time.
- Take a thoughtful approach to how negative health information about foods is shared.

Keeping these six guidelines in mind, you should also tailor your approach to sharing nutritional information, and the language you use to share it, depending on your child's age. Here are some guidelines for how to talk to kids about the nutritional benefits of different foods by age:

Ages 0–2

At these young ages, I encourage you to focus on very simple concepts related to food and nutrition, like the words for foods and naming the colors of foods. These are the earliest building blocks for beginning to teach your child that different foods do different things in our bodies.

Ages 3–5

When talking to kids about food during the preschool years, you still want to work with highly simplified concepts. The underlying goal of conversations at this age is to provide kids with information without an emotional spin. You might say, "Corn gives you energy, plus the yellow color comes from two chemicals that can keep your eyes healthy for a long time," or "Eggs can help your body build strong muscles."

By the time kids are in school, attending birthday parties, and participating in activities, they will begin to understand that hyperpalatable foods are different from other foods. They may be given these foods as special treats or rewards by other people. Their friends will make a big deal out of them, and of course, they taste way different! Kids know they are different. We don't have to make a big deal out of that fact, but we also don't have to pretend that they are the same. An important part of protecting your child's relationship with food and their body at this stage is teaching them that hyperpalatable foods are a *good* part of life and that it's healthy for us to include them in our diet *sometimes.*

Here are some scripts for specific food situations and questions that may come up during the preschool years:

> *In a situation where you want to label a hyperpalatable food:* "Candy has energy in it. Some foods do a lot of things in our bodies; some foods do a few things. Candy does a few things, and we eat it for fun. Eating for fun is important for us!"

> *Your child is asking for candy (or another food) when you aren't serving it:* "Candy isn't on the menu right now. Here's what is available. We'll have some candy after we visit Grandma."

> *Your child asks for a food and you are willing to include it:* "Cookies give us quick energy. Let's have it with a cheese stick to add some long energy."

A food doesn't make a balanced meal: "Cereal is an energy food. It gives us quick energy that lasts a short time. We're going to also have apples and peanut butter with this, because they give us energy that lasts a long time."

A food isn't what it seems: "This candy is called 'fruit snacks' because it's in the shape of fruit, but it's not fruit!"

Your child asks if a dessert is good for them or if it's "healthy": "Ice cream can help build our bones a little bit, and it's healthy for us to eat foods for fun. All foods can be healthy."

Parent agrees to serve a dessert after a child asks for it, but later in the day: "Sure, we'll have candy after lunch."

Parent wants to stress the importance of dental health without demonizing sweets: "We had candy, so it's important we brush our teeth!"

Ages 5–11

As kids get older and enter elementary school, they can handle more in-depth information about food and nutrition. They may start bringing home questions and comments about food from interacting with other kids and adults. They can also build on the idea that foods do things in their bodies and that they do more than one thing at a time, while still maintaining a morally neutral perspective. Your child will also be more aware of what they are hearing around them. They may wonder what "calories" are or hear that foods are bad if they have a lot of "fat" in them. They may also pick up the common message that "the more protein, the better," even though it's not always true.

Some of the messages that you want to convey to your kids at this age are more or less the same as when they were preschoolers, but you may expand a little bit, saying things like, "Bread is made out of grains. Grains can be white or brown, they give us energy, and they help us poop," or "A 'calorie' is a measurement of energy. We need energy for everything we do. Calories tell us how much energy we get from this food."

Here are some scripts for specific food situations and questions that may come up during the elementary school years:

A food doesn't make a balanced meal: "Cereal is a quick energy food. It runs out before lunchtime. That's why we serve it with a protein food, to help us stay full until lunchtime. What protein food would you like to add?"

A food isn't what it seems: "Would you like fruit snacks candy in your lunch?"

[*At a different time:*] "Look at this package. The company wants people to think this candy is fruit. I wonder why."

Your child asks if a dessert is good for them or if it's "healthy": "What do you mean by 'healthy'?"

There's a food parents will not buy: "That's not on the list."

"We're not going to buy this food because we buy foods when we [like the taste / like the way it makes our bodies feel / it's an important part of our culture]. That's important to me, and this food doesn't fit that description. We give companies our money for foods. When we buy foods, we tell companies what we want."

"Different families buy different things. We don't buy [X food], but [Y food] is one that our family buys."

Someone tells your child their food is unhealthy: "Different foods do different things in your body. Some foods do a lot of things;

some foods are mostly for fun. That food is mostly for fun. What would happen if we never ate fun foods? What would happen if we only ate fun foods?"

Your child's friend tells them that a food they're eating is "bad," "toxic," or "poisonous": "What do you think they meant by that? I wonder how they know if something is toxic or poisonous."

"I wonder where your friend got that information. That's actually not accurate."

Serving a new food: "This is [[name of new food]]. Here's a small piece for you to look at."

Parent needs to eat differently: "Everyone's body is different. Different bodies sometimes need different foods. This is the food that my body needs right now."

Your child's school does not allow sugary foods: "Sometimes some foods are good for some places and not for others. We don't send nuts, candy, or really messy foods to school. But we do eat all those things at home. [[X sugary food]] is not one that we send to school."

Someone tells your child that foods are categorized as "healthy" or "unhealthy": "It's healthy for us to eat cupcakes. Also, if we ate too many cupcakes, that would be unhealthy."

"What about peanuts? They are not safe for your friend with allergies, but they are safe for you. So are peanuts 'healthy' or 'unhealthy'?"

"This activity seems tricky! How do we know if a food is 'healthy' or 'unhealthy' when all foods are important and do different things in our bodies?"

[Your child may not have an answer, and that's okay! This exercise is about getting them thinking.]

Ages 12–18 (though adults benefit, too!)

Older children can begin to think more critically, and this is an appropriate time to start addressing some of the "negative" information they have been hearing about certain foods. They will need your guidance to help make sense of what they are hearing as they grow.

Some parents feel very strongly that sharing any negative information about foods will hurt a child's relationship with food, regardless of their age. While there is not sufficient evidence to uphold that assumption for typically developing kids, I respect the preference.

If a child is overly concerned about food or is highly anxious, or someone in the household struggles with disordered eating, sticking to the positive may be a good starting point for practicing curiosity. You might say things like, "There are different types of fat. For example, avocados have a lot of monounsaturated fat. This type of fat can reduce inflammation in your heart." Or, "Leafy greens have prebiotics and lots of other good things in them. They feed the helpful microbes in your gut. Good microbes are an important part of your immune system; they make vitamins for you and help you have a healthy brain."

Here are some scripts for specific food situations and questions that may come up in the tween and teen years:

A food doesn't make a balanced meal: "Cereal gives us quick energy. That means your body breaks it down into energy quickly, then your body burns through it, and you end up tired and hungry. To make the energy last, we need foods with fat and protein. Have you thought about one of these options?"

A food isn't what it seems: "Companies use words on a box to try to get people to buy their products. You'll see them on most food packages. Fruit snacks are a great candy. But companies want parents to think it's fruit. . . . I wonder how the company makes money from this."

Your child is wondering why you are buying fewer hyperpalatable foods: "Companies work really hard to make us want to buy certain foods. They don't care that too many of those foods aren't good for our health. I don't want to give those companies as much of my money, so I'm going to add in some different foods when I shop now. We'll still have fun foods sometimes, and I also want to try out some new snack ideas for us to add into our diet."

"I realized our family isn't eating enough fiber/protein/veggies/nutrients. We got into the habit of eating so many 'fun' foods we haven't been meeting our nutrient needs. So, I'm buying more foods to help us get what we need to think clearly, grow, and feel strong and less of the foods we've been eating too much of. We'll still have them, though."

Parent agrees to buy/serve requested hyperpalatable foods: "Here are the cookies you wanted to go with your snack."

"Sure, I'll add chips to the shopping list for this week."

Your child asks if a dessert is good for them or healthy, or starts talking about desserts being unhealthy: "There are foods that do the same things, but to different degrees. One term for this is *nutrient density*. This doesn't make a food good or bad; it just gives us information that we can use. It's important for us to eat all kinds of foods so that we get all the nutrition that we need."

"Eating dessert is healthy. Eating too many desserts is unhealthy. We have to make sure we get all the nutrients we need from other foods like protein, fiber, vitamins, and minerals. We know we're eating too many desserts if we feel sick or if we can't eat enough of the other nutrients we need."

"I wonder why dessert is unhealthy." [They might give you the chance to talk about weight stigma, weight-loss diets, food myths, or other topics.]

There's a food parents will not buy: "I choose to spend my money on certain foods for certain reasons. I don't want to support this company's product line based on what they are doing. Every person gets to make the choices that are important to them. You are starting to spend money on food, too, so you can make your own choices about what you will buy and what messages you want to send with your purchases."

"This food has more sugar than is helpful for us. We enjoy lots of other foods with sugar, so I prefer not to buy this particular one."

"Energy drinks are not safe for kids/teens. They have too much caffeine and other substances."

Your child starts to think some foods are "bad," "toxic," or "poisonous": "Who gets to decide which foods are good and which foods are bad?"

"People are using the word *toxic* to describe a lot of foods. Which foods haven't been labeled 'toxic'?"

"Let's find out the facts. This food is definitely not toxic, but there's something people don't like about it." [You can explore whether it is an identity mascot food, whether the information is false, or whether it's tied to diet culture in some way.]

IF YOUR CHILD TAKES AN UNHEALTHY INTEREST IN NUTRITION INFORMATION OR TRACKING

If your child is perfectionistic, obsesses about what foods are doing in their body, refuses most just-for-fun foods, worries about their weight, or is having mental health struggles, it's important to think critically about the nutritional information you share with them. As we discussed earlier, these could be early indicators of disordered eating. If your child exhibits any of these traits, it may be helpful to avoid discussing negative nutritional information, instead reinforcing that it is okay to eat all foods. But even if you emphasize that all foods are okay to eat, kids with these tendencies will of course hear that some foods are "unhealthy" outside of the home. In this case, it may be helpful to address this head-on with them by saying, "Foods do different things in our bodies, and some foods have less nutrition. Some people say that makes those foods 'unhealthy.' But it is important for our health to eat all foods, even foods that are just for enjoyment and fun. If we worry a lot about what is in food and have rules about not eating certain foods, that is unhealthy for us. Our family will continue to eat all foods."

As a side note: If you struggle with disordered eating yourself, and having conversations about nutrition challenges your mental health, give yourself permission to skip them. You do not have to talk to your child about food if you don't want to. Your mental health gets priority.

A teacher recently approached me for advice on implementing nutrition education in their all-girls school to help the students know how to fuel their bodies properly and eat a balanced diet. She was concerned because she learned that among the fourth-grade girls, it was becoming "cool" to skip lunch, and she wanted to make sure the girls' relationships with their bodies were kept in mind. The school was already doing an excellent job of providing a variety of foods at lunchtime, positive food exposures, and positive food information. After speaking with her more, it became apparent that the girls likely had all the nutrition information they needed, but what they most needed to know was that it is healthy to be able to enjoy just-for-fun foods. My suggestion for this school was to have an educational unit on desserts, where they learn to make desserts from different countries and then enjoy those foods together.

I was once interviewed on a podcast where the host told me she had been training her daughter from a young age to read labels and decide if something had "too much sugar," which led to an awkward pause on my part while I tried to figure out how to respond. Although this kind of training might be helpful for children with certain health conditions, it can also put a burden on a child to follow the "right" rules when it comes to eating and it will likely decrease enjoyment of eating and choosing foods. Tracking the sugar content in food is often emblematic of diet culture and disordered eating, and it's not a healthy activity for children to be participating in unless they have a medical reason.

Keep in mind that how we talk about food with our kids is something that's meant to change over time. It's not something we need to obsess over and it's certainly not something that is going to ruin our kids if we don't "do it right." If we can counteract the loud external good/bad and hyperpalatable food messages with age-appropriate messages of our own, we are doing our part to arm kids with the information they need to eat a varied diet, take care of their health, and have a positive relationship with their bodies.

5

EAT WHAT NOURISHES US

"I *feel so drained and tired all the time . . . My forearms and wrists hurt . . . my mood is down . . .*" I was sitting in the doctor's office when my kids were one and three, giving my doctor a list of symptoms.

"*Well, you've got a desk job and two little kids. That's sometimes just how it is at this stage of life,*" my doctor told me.

A year later, I still couldn't shake the feeling that my symptoms were about more than two little kids and a desk job. I was *so* exhausted and out of sorts, but I couldn't get my doctor to hear me. I found a specialized registered dietitian who ordered some blood work and told me to eat a lot more vegetables (everyone can use a reminder now and then) because I needed the nutrients. Adding more veggies to my diet did help a bit. But when the blood tests came back, she reported, "Your B12 is low. You'll feel a lot better if we fix that." I had pernicious anemia (caused by not having enough B12), and when she helped me resolve it, my life completely changed for the better (and I finally understood how people had the energy to take their toddlers places). Nutrition in general—and specific nutrients—matter for us and for our kids. And while there are plenty of other things that our bodies also need to thrive, eating what nourishes us, which is the fifth pillar, is an essential piece of the puzzle.

Parents ask me questions every day about what their children need to eat to be healthy. They ask what will happen if their kids don't eat vegetables. They ask if they are slowly poisoning their kids with sugar, processed foods, anything served in plastic, even water. Parents wonder if they should be worried about certain ingredients in foods or if it is worthwhile to buy organic produce or the "better version" of various foods (whatever that means to you). They wonder if any of it matters at all. What to feed our kids feels more complicated than ever because there is so much information being thrown at us. We need a simple system that we can use to evaluate the health and food info coming our way, so that we can decide what to pay attention to and what to disregard when it comes to helping our kids nourish their bodies. We don't want them to have nutritional deficiencies, but we also don't want our heads to explode from how complicated nutrition seems to have become.

THE HEALTH IMPACT TIERS

Eating what nourishes us begins by knowing how to make decisions about what our bodies, and what our kids' bodies, need. It's also about determining what is doable, practically speaking, for your family, without obsessing over every ingredient you're feeding your child.

To aid busy parents in this effort, I have created two separate tools for determining what is important to be feeding your child right now, depending on how into the weeds you want to get on specific health needs. The first tool, which I call the Health Impact Tiers, is for parents looking for more detailed information on practical nutrition. If you have no interest in spending time in the nutritional weeds, that's cool, too. Feel free to jump to the next section, where I offer my Nutrition Basics version of this tool.

Your child's nutrition *is* important. Nutrition matters. But not *everything* you hear about nutrition matters, not everything that matters about nutrition matters to *your* child, and not everything that matters to your child has the same *level* of importance. Although it can be okay for parents to be really into nutrition, your child will most likely be just fine without you going down a rabbit hole of child nutrition and making it your part-time job. No one should feel guilty if they don't have the time for or the interest in making nutrition a focal point of their parenting.

My Health Impact Tiers are designed to help you prioritize what nutritional issues will matter most for your child, and they're a tool you can refer to if you're ever feeling overwhelmed or confused by a feeding decision. All the health tiers are important, and the tiers at the top have the broadest impact on children's overall health, likely influencing the tiers below them.

Tier 1: *Living*—The essential food actions to take to protect your child

Tier 2: *Growing*—The food elements necessary for basic growth

Tier 3: *Thriving*—The essentials necessary for maintaining overall health

Tier 4: *Optimizing*—The actions to take to make sure all your child's nutrient needs are being met

Tier 5: *Fine-Tuning*—Little tweaks to support optimal health

Tier 6: *Individualizing*—Food choices based on emerging areas of research, food philosophies, personal preference, and identity.

It is most important to focus on the first three tiers, to ensure that your child is getting the essential nourishment that they need. But you don't have to do all the things in every tier perfectly to reap health benefits for your child. Nutrition is nuanced—through a practice of curiosity, you may find that for *your* kid, something in a lower tier has a very broad impact. Understanding this hierarchy, even if you don't follow it exactly, will help you make informed choices for yourself, your child, and your family. This is not a quest for perfection. It's a guide for practical decision-making.

For most of us, there will be some seasons of life where we're handling all the tiers like a champ and other seasons when we can barely handle the big stuff. I created the tiers for that reason. Maybe last year you tackled it all, but this year, you're in survival mode. Which tiers matter most when you're trying to get through a rough spot? Living and Growing. If things lighten up a little, you can focus on Living, Growing, and Thriving. As you have more capacity, you can work on the nutrition elements in tiers 4 through 6.

TIER 1: LIVING

Allergies, medical conditions, choking hazards, food recalls, food safety, energy

Food allergies, such medical conditions as celiac disease or diabetes, choking hazards—these are first line. They always get priority attention. Additionally, if there's a food recall, pay attention. And make sure you know the basics of food safety, the most important of which are to keep cold foods cold and hot foods hot until eating, cook food thoroughly to a safe temperature, wash raw produce thoroughly, and put leftovers away promptly and eat them within five days. No parent loves earning the "survived a round of family food poisoning" badge, not to mention the fact that food poisoning can leave lingering effects, such as compromised gut health. Additionally, energy is the foundation of living. Kids need enough calories. This is why we advocate for a strong nutrition safety net (government programs that ensure access to food—in the US, that's SNAP, national school meal programs, WIC, and more), use food assistance for our families if we ever qualify for it, and feed our kids whatever they will eat if their eating challenges are preventing them from getting enough calories.

TIER 2: GROWING

Protein, food reactions, deficiencies, movement, sleep

There are many elements necessary to ensure a child's healthy growth. Some are individualized, but others are universal. All kids need enough protein to grow. If a child has an obvious negative reaction to food dyes, additives, or foods, such as lactose, those items need to be removed from their diet. Nutrient deficiencies, like iron or vitamin D, must be resolved as soon as possible.

Most kids get plenty of protein and often need less protein than many people think—requirements are based on their weight. Here's a general range per size and age:

- A 28-pound (13 kg) toddler: 13–17 g of protein per day
- A 45-pound (20 kg) elementary-age child: 20–31 g of protein per day
- A 70-pound (32 kg) elementary-age child: 30–49 g of protein per day
- A 90-pound (41 kg) tween: 39–53 g of protein per day
- A 120-pound (55 kg) teen: 46–71 g of protein per day

Toddlers and preschoolers may eat like birds on certain days, and parents might worry they aren't getting enough protein. But their protein needs are pretty small! There are 16 g of protein in two cups of milk, 12 g in two eggs, and about 14 g in a peanut butter and jelly sandwich (depending on which bread and how much peanut butter). Protein is in almost all foods, including vegetables and grains.

If you have a concern about your child's protein intake, especially if they don't eat many protein foods, spend a few days tracking how much they are eating. Otherwise, there is no need to get wrapped up in this. Serve a protein food with all meals and snacks (unless serving them with a snack will ruin their appetite for dinner), let them ask for more if you have it available, and leave it at that. If you do see that your child really is not getting enough protein, you may need to change what you are offering. That may mean not offering fruit or low-protein veggies as often, or having snacks comprised primarily of protein foods, such as hummus on high-protein toast or bagel, hard-boiled eggs, chicken or tuna salad sandwiches, or cheese sticks. Just make sure the protein is primarily coming from foods, not from a lot of protein powders, drinks, or bars (having a small amount of your high-protein smoothie or bite of your protein bar is fine and giving a tween or teen a protein bar is not a problem). While protein supplements may be helpful in some situations, most kids, even kids in sports, can get all the protein they need from food, and they risk getting too much when you add powders, drinks, and bars if they already eat a balanced diet. If you think your child is getting too much protein and they eat a lot of animal products, consider swapping out some animal proteins for some plant sources of protein like beans, nuts, or seeds. Plant sources of protein are a great way to get protein and provide nutrition such as fiber, color pigments, vitamins, and minerals, which animal sources of protein can sometimes crowd out.

Movement and sleep are also tier 2 elements. It may seem strange to include movement and sleep in a chapter about nutrition. But when it comes to keeping our kids healthy, these are equally or even more important than what our kids eat and are associated with all the benefits that you hope nutrition will bring to your child. If your child isn't getting enough sleep, no amount of good nutrition is going to keep them healthy, and it may be harder for them to hear their typical hunger and fullness cues. Movement—whether it is walking, playing on the playground, biking, dancing, or competing in a sport—gets their blood flowing, which brings nutrients and oxygen to all the little parts of their bodies. Plus, movement helps kids work up an appetite, and hungry kids are more likely to eat what you make for dinner (my source for this is thirteen years of life experience feeding children).

TIER 3: THRIVING

Fat, fiber, water, and avoiding high-heavy-metal foods, processed meats, sugar-sweetened beverages, and baby rice products

If a child is meeting their protein and energy needs, then you've achieved stability and can now think beyond just survival.

Kids need fats, especially unsaturated fats and plenty of omega-3 fatty acids, and we want to make sure they are getting these fats from a variety of sources. Foods such as avocado, nuts and seeds, nut or seed butters, fatty fish (like salmon, trout, and sardines), and plant-based oils, such as olive oil, are great fat sources to add to their meals. Foods high in protein usually have fat as well, so if kids are getting enough protein and a fat source is used in cooking, then they are getting enough fat in their diet. One way to help your child get enough omega-3 fatty acids is by serving them low-mercury fatty fish twice a week.

Next, fiber is a big deal. Protein gets the most attention in the press, but fiber is the one that *needs* the most attention. Fiber comes from fruit, vegetables (including beans, lentils, and starchy veggies), whole grains, nuts, and/or seeds. If your child is getting enough fiber, that is going to be protective of many things. Not only does it help prevent constipation, which is a common issue in children, but it feeds the "good guys" (helpful microbes) in the gut. Fiber and your child's gut health impact your child's blood sugar, immune system, cancer risk, mental health, risk of heart disease, inflammation, ability to absorb nutrients, digestion, and more. Ninety-five percent of children are *not* meeting fiber recommendations in the United States, so unless you know your child is getting enough, I wouldn't worry about exactly how many grams your child is eating and instead just focus on adding *more*. See the appendix for fiber needs by age.

The next thing is water. Help your child drink water as their primary drink. Fluid is essential, especially if you're increasing a child's fiber intake. Increasing fiber without fluid will result in constipation. Kids can also drink milk (animal or plant-based), but that shouldn't be their primary liquid, as it can crowd out nutritional variety from other foods, contribute to picky eating, and lead to kids drinking their meals. Avoid sugar-sweetened beverages for your child, too. This might sound like an extreme recommendation, but sugar-sweetened beverages are associated with higher risk of many chronic diseases (from cancer to heart disease). The drinks themselves are hard on kids' bodies, and by avoiding them we prevent them from developing a habit of drinking sugary drinks and getting used to the hypersweet flavor. There may be specific instances when sugar-sweetened beverages serve a particular purpose, such as in the case of a sports drink or chocolate milk for sports performance or recovery. They also may play an important social or cultural role, or be necessary to solve a nutrition problem, but in general we want to be thoughtful about offering these beverages. Juice is a bit different. There are a few caveats—don't give your infant juice if they are under age one (unless you're following medical advice) and delay introducing juice until age two or older to prevent your child from getting used to hypersweet drink flavors (as well as reducing possible exposure to heavy metals in the juice). After they've been exposed to juice, though, you can offer it sometimes and in diluted form or in small portions. Juice can be helpful for meeting micronutrient needs, helping kids take medications, treating dehydration, or treating and preventing constipation, so it shouldn't be completely off the table for all kids from a nutrition standpoint. It has a place. But even if juice is helpful in some circumstances, water can still be the primary drink.

For some families, drinking filtered water is part of thriving. If you know or suspect your water is contaminated by nearby factories, farming, insufficient water regulations, or old pipes, then filtering your water (ideally with a reverse osmosis filter or multistage carbon filter, but if not, the most thorough one you can get) is important. In the US, public water utilities have been required to send water reports to all customers annually. Contact your local utility company to find out if they send these water reports, which should include chemical levels, the national regulation levels, and whether the water ever had chemicals over the regulation levels. You can look at your water report and decide whether it makes sense to filter your water.

Finally, there are a few foods to avoid because they can be very high in heavy metals. One is high-mercury fish, such as king mackerel, marlin, orange roughy, shark, swordfish, tilefish, and bigeye tuna. Salmon and sardines are examples of good low-mercury fatty fish to serve kids.

Spices and imported candy containing spices are sometimes contaminated by lead during the production process. I don't want you to think spices are "dangerous" and to stop serving them, because spices are so important—they make food taste good, they have many health benefits when used in cooking, and they are used in culinary medicine. Please still use spices in your cooking, even for your young kids! Just be mindful of where you are getting them. For spices, contamination is more likely to occur in discount, small, or non–name brands that have less oversight over the production process. Imported candy with spices in it and bulk spice bins are also more likely to have lead contamination. If you use spices routinely, buy name-brand or bigger-store-brand spices if possible, not in little packets (these packets have recently been sources of contaminated spices in broad recalls, such as a massive cinnamon recall), and vary the brands that you buy, because heavy metal levels can vary among different batches of spices that are produced for the same brand. This is the only time in this book you will hear me outright recommend you buy a brand name or bigger-store-brand name.

Processed meats are red meat, poultry, and fish that have been salted, fermented, smoked, cured, or undergone other processes. They are classified as carcinogenic. There is enough data that researchers are confident they cause colon cancer. It has not been determined if they cause other types of cancer. Researchers don't fully know which part(s) of processing cause cancer (the nitrates, chemicals in smoke, heme iron in the meat, chemicals created when the meat is cooked at high temperatures, etc.). More research has been done on processed red meats than processed poultry products. Eating processed meat doesn't mean someone will definitely get cancer, but it increases their risk of getting colorectal cancer. The existing research shows that the more processed meat someone consumes, the higher their risk. Red meat is also associated with colorectal cancer (and others), but it has only been classified as "probably carcinogenic" because more research is needed to determine if it's the cause. Red meat is tricky, because it can be an excellent source of iron and other nutrients for kids (or parents) who are low on these nutrients, even while it may carry risk. If colon cancer runs in your family or if you have other concerns, you might consider being especially vigilant about reducing how much red meat your family eats. If not, you might still consider how much you eat. Our family takes a moderate approach at this time as we acknowledge our family's nutrient needs, and we eat red meat a few times a month and limit processed meats.

The final foods to avoid are processed baby rice products, such as rice cereal, teething biscuits, and puffs, because they can contain high levels of arsenic. My recommendations do not apply to rice itself. You can still feed rice to babies, and rice as a staple food for families is fine. This only pertains to processed rice products. There are easy alternatives available made from other grains, like oats.

TIER 4: OPTIMIZING

Variety, micronutrients, filtered water, added sugars, sodium, saturated fat

Here is where you might begin to fine-tune your child's diet to make sure they're getting all the little things they need and not getting too much of whatever they don't need.

To start, consider vitamins and minerals, also known as *micronu-*

trients. These are the chemicals your body needs to work properly. If a child is eating enough protein (including animal sources) and energy and is getting enough fat and fiber from foods, there's a good chance they will be getting all the micronutrients they need (if a child does not consume animal sources of protein, then supplementation of B12 is necessary). This is especially true if a child is getting *variety*. Variety means different kinds of foods in the same food group. Different types of proteins, different types of veggies and fruits and grains. The more the merrier. If you want to add more variety, you can start slowly and realistically by adding one new food a week or a month.

Iron and calcium are the two nutrients that parents ask me about the most. All kids need iron, and babies, toddlers, and teen girls are especially at risk of deficiency, so make sure to include plenty of iron-rich foods in their diets. The foods include fish, poultry, meat, beans, leafy greens, and iron-fortified foods. The trick for iron is to serve iron-rich foods with foods that have vitamin C, such as fruits and veggies. (The appendix has more information about daily iron needs. Calcium recommendations vary widely internationally, and you can also find those in the appendix.)

At this point, making sure your child is getting a variety of colors and food categories will help them get all the micronutrients they need. If you've already been working on adequate fiber, and kids are getting that through whole grains, fruits, vegetables, and nuts/seeds, your child is already on their way to getting these nutrients. Supplements are usually necessary to meet recommendations for vitamin D, especially if you live in a northern climate or your child is not outside very often.

At the optimizing stage, we're not just thinking about how to get a child to eat more fiber in any way possible—now we're thinking about which sources of fiber will also provide the nutrients that a child is low in. Foods all have many nutrients in them, and most of them include protein, vitamins, minerals, and other compounds, but here are some specific foods and the nutrients they get attention for:

- Beans for minerals, including some calcium
- Dark green, leafy, and deeply colored veggies for vitamins and minerals
- Orange veggies for vitamin A
- Nuts and seeds for vitamin E and minerals, including some calcium
- Fruit and bell peppers for vitamin C and to help with iron absorption
- Organ meats and fatty fish for vitamin B12, vitamin A, iron, vitamin D, and omega-3 fatty acids
- Fortified foods, such as soy milk fortified with calcium
- Canned fish with bones for highly absorbable calcium
- Dairy for calcium

Filtered water is in this optimizing tier, even though it doesn't necessarily apply to all families. As I've mentioned, if you know your water quality isn't meeting regulations, then filtered water is part of Thriving. But even if you haven't heard anything about your water, filtering it might be helpful. It is my hope that the US government will continue to add regulations regarding allowable levels of chemicals in water as they learn more about the presence of various chemicals and what their effects are in the body. However, new regulations take time to implement and are sometimes affected by politics. For example, in early 2024, the government released a new regulation for PFAS ("forever chemicals") in drinking water—setting "maximum contaminant levels" for six of them (there are thousands)—due to the substantial evidence of the harm they cause to human health. However, after a change in administration, the priorities were changed. The regulation for four of the PFAS is expected to be rescinded, so it's unclear if/when those PFAS will be regulated in water. In the meantime, the chemicals are in many water supplies. So, if you can remove them on your own with a reverse osmosis, multistage carbon filter, or other water filters, you are effectively implementing the regulation for your family.

Next, there are a few things to keep an eye on reducing, specifically added sugar, sodium, and saturated fat, which kids eat too much of. Currently, over 60 percent of children ages two to four, 80 percent of children ages five to thirteen, and over 70 percent of children ages fourteen and older are eating more added sugars than recommended. As a rule, we want kids to eat 24 g or less of added sugars per day. Too many added sugars can make foods hyperpalatable and thus make "normal" foods taste less exciting; crowd out nutrient-dense foods; suppress the immune system; contribute to cavities, unhealthy blood lipids, and inflammation; and lead to grumpy kids when their sugar highs wear off.

Keep in mind that this is a tier 4 concern. If you've focused on the first three tiers, you may have already crowded out some added sugars from foods or sugar-sweetened beverages. This is a great time to focus on who your child is, since added sugars can help get some kids to eat enough food, address picky eating, or make fibrous foods tastier and more attractive. Becoming obsessive about sugar management is not the goal (and it's no help to parents' mental health!). Instead, focus on being aware of and intentional about added sugar consumption.

Next, over 90 percent of kids are eating too much sodium. Sodium is essential to be healthy, but too much can stress the kidneys and make high blood pressure more likely. Like added sugars, sodium can make foods hyperpalatable and make normal foods taste less exciting. But also like added sugars, adding sodium can make normal foods taste better, which can be helpful in many cases, such as picky eating and low appetite.

Finally, 80 percent or more of children up to age eighteen are eating more saturated fat than recommended, which contributes to the risk of heart disease and stroke. Saturated fat comes from animal proteins, including dairy, but like the other items that make foods hyperpalatable, bacon or cheese have also been known to help kids eat more of whatever food they are in. That may serve a purpose in some cases for getting kids to eat certain foods.

Added sugars, sodium, and saturated fat are often found in the same foods. To address all three, consider offering fewer sweet products (candy, sweetened yogurt, desserts, ready-to-eat cereal) or high-sodium foods (pizza—the top contributor to sodium intake—salty snacks, processed or brined meats, or high-sodium soups). Think about delaying your child's introduction to foods with added sugars and sodium for as long as possible. Finally, eating less fast food and cooking at home whenever possible can help decrease sugar, sodium, and saturated fat intake.

TIER 5: FINE-TUNING

Phytochemicals, probiotics, dietary plant diversity, artificial dyes, heavy metals, processed versus unprocessed foods

If you and your child have tiers 1 through 4 covered, you are doing very well! I know this is a lot to juggle with everything you are dealing with as a parent day to day. While the topics under tier 5 are secondary to those covered in the other tiers, they tend to get more attention in the media because they make for good headlines. They are important, but they don't have as broad of an impact on the health of children as tiers 1 through 4.

Phytochemicals. These are plant compounds that do great things in our bodies. They can be antioxidants and fight off some of the molecules that do damage in our bodies. They are associated with such health benefits as decreased risk of cancer and dementia. Deeper-color fruits and vegetables, especially blue/purple (but all the other colors, including white, too), berries, and cruciferous veggies (cabbage, broccoli, cauliflower, collards, kale, etc.) all get a lot of attention for their plant compounds. Remember, though, all plants have compounds, so they are all great. If you've already Optimized (tier 4), then your child is likely getting many phytochemicals.

Probiotics. Probiotics are the "little guys" (sounds cuter than *microbes*) in the gut that make vitamin K for us, interact with our brains in a good way, help us absorb the right things, and fight off bad microbes that will make us sick. Kids can get them from foods that have been fermented. Here are some examples: yogurt with "live active cultures," fermented pickles, sauerkraut, and kimchi (the ones with the little guys are refrigerated), tempeh, miso, and kefir. These little guys need fiber to eat, so incorporating these foods into a diet that already contains fiber can be great for your child's gut health. Different strains of probiotics can also have specific health indications.

Dietary plant diversity. Researchers have observed that the more plant foods we consume, the more diverse our gut microbiome, meaning that we will have a wider variety of microbes living in our gut. This is a good thing. Specifically, the emerging research in this area is based on people consuming thirty or more plant foods per week, such as fruits, veggies, nuts, or seeds. Aiming for forty, fifty, or more plant foods is also great! That's often a tall order. There's a reason this is in the "refining" tier—it's a lot to keep track of, many people don't have access to this much variety, it can be expensive, and you have to have a kid who will actually eat it. If it all aligns for you, though, go for it! This can be a great way to nurture your child's health. And you might already be further ahead than you think you are. Take a family who eats quinoa, brown rice, oats, popcorn, and wheat over the course of the week. That's five. Their weekly menu often includes tomato sauce, cucumbers, carrots, broccoli, bell peppers, cauliflower, celery, sweet potatoes and golden potatoes, onions, garlic, and lettuce. That's twelve. They also eat protein veggies like black beans, garbanzo beans, and peas. That's three. They have lemons for cooking and serve applesauce, bananas, clementines, frozen blueberries, raisins, and another fruit like kiwis. That's another seven. And they routinely eat chopped walnuts on their oatmeal, and peanut butter and sunflower seed butter sandwiches. That brings them to thirty different plant foods.

Artificial dyes. Artificial dyes can negatively impact some kids' behavior. If you know your child has an obvious adverse reaction to artificial dyes, this issue falls under "food reactions" in tier 2 alongside protein and energy. If your child doesn't have an obvious reaction to food dyes, you might be curious about their effect given the recent media and political attention to this issue, which makes it sound like most if not all children react to food dyes.

If you've been following the tiers in order of priority, you're already working on reducing added sugar and salty snacks and increasing your child's fiber intake. Just by doing these things, your child's exposure to artificial dyes will be limited. If you'd like to know if your child is affected by dyes, you can do an experiment where you remove artificial dyes from their diet for a few weeks and then return them to their normal diet for a few weeks. Note your observations. Do this twice and get feedback on your child's behavior from two other people, including one who doesn't know you are testing food dyes. This prevents biases from clouding your observations. You can use this procedure for any diet changes you want to test with your child.

I've included dyes in this tier because there is enough reliable evidence to suggest that the behavior of some children is affected by dyes and that some kids may be consuming more than the safe levels of certain dyes. If you notice behavior changes when your child consumes food dye, you may choose to move this issue to tier 2, Growing. If you don't notice behavior changes, this topic drops down to tier 6, Individualizing. You don't have to get wrapped up in this issue. My husband and I suspect that one of our kids is sensitive to dyes, but we haven't explored it much. At the same time, because we are focusing on the higher tiers, we know that he doesn't have much exposure to dyes. If we have a choice, we choose foods without artificial colors. We take an aware but laid-back approach to this.

Heavy metals. We already talked about the heavy hitters of heavy metals—the ones that I recommend everyone think about and avoid—like high-mercury fish. But every other week, there's a new report coming out about a variety of heavy metals in foods like root veggies, baby food (homemade and otherwise), seeds, rice, chocolate, and more. There seem to be countless reports and countless foods with heavy metals in them. This is because the ground has heavy metals and so does water, and plants take in the water. Heavy metals can also be unintentionally added to foods through food processing. These reports aren't baseless, although they are usually presented out of context and make everything sound unnecessarily alarmist. We do want kids to get as little of these metals as possible, so it may be helpful in some cases to pay attention. I recommend referring to the section below, "The Five Questions for Food Headlines," to decide whether it's a priority for you to change your child's diet based on the latest headlines.

TIER 6: INDIVIDUALIZING

Additives, pesticides, organic foods, contaminants

Now we get into the *most* divisive and emotionally charged topics, ones that are also widely reported and discussed in the media, despite difference in interpretations of how they affect our health. For some topics, such as additives, pesticides on foods, and organic diets, data and research on the short- and long-term health effects isn't as strong as headlines make it sound. That means the relevant research is largely observational (if it even exists) and sometimes conflicts. When it comes to these topics, parents often want a definitive answer because the headlines are unsettling. "Is organic food better for my child?" (I'm sorry, I cannot with any certainty tell you it is.) "Are food additives, like aspartame or monk fruit extract, eaten in realistic portions, going to increase my child's risk of cancer?" (Again, I can't tell you they will or won't.) Some people are *very* confident in their interpretations of the research, whether they believe that all additives are toxic or completely fine. But for every expert who believes they are right on these topics, there is another expert with an opposite conclusion who also has research references to back up their stance. The truth is that both sides can be right in certain ways. For example, it might be possible for a specific artificial ingredient to increase some people's risk of colon cancer, but not for most people, and not for any other kind of cancer.

It might also be possible for organic food to make a difference for specific children with one uncommon trait and have no effect on all the other kids.

As always, I support whatever food choices and beliefs are important to you, and I'll support you if you decide to take a stance on these issues (even if I won't tell you you're absolutely right). There are some pitfalls to be aware of in tier 6, however. First, we should be mindful of the amount of anxiety that focusing on these issues can cause. Second, taking a strong stance on some of these issues can make people who don't have the ability or option to work on them (those who can't afford organic groceries, for example) feel baselessly guilty or inadequate. Third, focusing too much on tier 6 can take our attention, resources, and effort away from the other tiers with the broadest impact. If you are focusing on the higher-priority tiers, your child is likely doing well. If you get caught up in tier 6 to the detriment of the other tiers, your child may be missing important elements in their diet that can have a lifelong impact. For example, if your child isn't eating enough fiber, putting your resources into purchasing organic hyperpalatable cookies isn't where the big health benefits (both long and short term) will be for your child. If you choose to stop serving foods you have heard are dangerous due to a specific additive, but your child doesn't have a replacement source of foods with those nutrients, you may be putting your child's health at risk. If a child who doesn't have a visible reaction to food dye isn't getting enough iron, neglecting the iron deficiency and instead putting that effort into finding dye-free foods is missing the forest for the trees.

Putting a large emphasis on tier 6 foods can also sometimes cause us to over- or underestimate benefits and risks. Becoming overly focused on "toxic additives," for example, might make it easier for us to fall prey to the enormous amount of food marketing pushing "clean" and "natural" foods without additives—even though these foods are often just hyperpalatable foods made in a different way. "Organic fruit gummies with only real ingredients" that are colored with beet extract instead of artificial food dye are still hyperpalatable foods marketed to children, associated with all the risks of sweet hyperpalatable foods—alterations to the brain reward system, overeating, crowding out other nutrients, and more—despite the fact that they are marketed as health food. I came across a new product recently: strips of dried fruit that could be licked and dipped into a small pouch of dried maple sugar. This product was reminiscent of a candy available when I was a child, it tasted like candy, and it was every bit a hyperpalatable food, regardless of descriptors like "organic," "natural," "real fruit," "healthy," and "no additives" on the box.

Don't get me wrong—this food is fun and tasty, and you may decide that it's one you want your kids to enjoy. There is also a whole "better swaps" movement, which involves swapping typical hyperpalatable or processed foods for "healthier alternatives" (without artificial additives). I'm all for an additive-free version of a favorite snack when available. However, let's recognize this movement for what it is: an incredibly lucrative food marketing campaign! If you are following the tier system, your child is already eating fewer hyperpalatable foods and the dyes or additives that come with them. And although I don't have data to back up my hypothesis, I have a concern that the better swaps movement is increasing the amount of hyperpalatable foods children eat, thereby crowding out nutritional variety and priming them for a long-term hyperpalatable food consumption. I think many parents have held back on purchasing foods because of concerns about hyperpalatability and additives, and now that they are told the new versions of the food are "healthier" with "no bad stuff" (as one brand puts it), they don't feel any reason to hold back.

A strong focus on the categories under Individualizing can also contribute to "good/bad/healthy/unhealthy" language surrounding food for parents and children as we discussed in the previous chapter. This tier comes with significant risks for children with the beginnings of disordered eating, fueling their black-and-white food mentality and restrictive eating. So, while tier 6 may be important for our sense of identity or our exploration of optimal health for our families, it's also the tier to which we need to bring the most curiosity and discernment. We need to be aware of how the information might affect our kids (or adults around us) and think about how we can foster our identity in a way that still allows us to be able to enjoy food without fear or letting it overtake all the other eating priorities in our lives.

THE NUTRITION BASICS

Maybe everything I've shared up to this point about the food tiers and specific nutrients is just too in the weeds for you. That's fine! I also have a shortcut version of the Health Impact Tiers systems that I developed, first for my family and then shared with the Kids Eat in Color community in *Real Easy Weekdays*. I created the Nutrition Basics as a quick-reference set of guidelines to use so that we don't have to constantly think about nutrition. It is also research-based, only less in depth, and it's a great way to plan meals when you're in a hurry. Remember: *This is a collection of actions to aim toward, not something to measure your success as a parent against*. The Nutrition Basics guidelines give us the goal of including the following in your daily meal plan:

- Protein and fats at all meals
- A veggie (which can be any vegetable, including potatoes, beans, or lentils) or fruit at every meal
- A red or orange and a dark green vegetable every day
- Some whole grains (not necessarily all whole grain; some can be refined) and/or starches throughout the day
- A variety of foods
- Water

The other side of that is that we want to limit the following items when possible:

- Sweets and salty snacks
- Meats and dairy high in saturated fats
- Processed meats
- Fast food
- Any sugary beverages

Some days, my family checks all the boxes, but plenty of days, we don't. Rather than looking at exactly what my kids eat each individual day, I think about how they are eating over the course of a week or month. The body stores many nutrients and has them ready to go when needed. Energy needs vary day to day. A day of poor eating isn't going to impact their overall health—it's what they eat over weeks and months that counts. It's also not reasonable to be thinking about micronutrients all the time. I don't have the brain space for that.

When I'm planning meals on the fly, I also like to use the following equation as a shortcut for creating balanced meals and snacks:

A Balanced Meal =

Protein + Fat + Color + Carbohydrate

Protein and fat are often combined in the same food, such as in tuna or hummus. "Color" is fruits and vegetables. When my kids were little, my little "goal" was "fruit and veggie at every meal." This was helpful because it made it more likely to get at least one of them on the kids' plates. I know other people who have little goals, too, like, "don't serve the same food twice in a day" or "serve a raw veggie and cooked veggie at dinner." If the idea of a goal like this stresses you out, you don't have to use one. If you find them helpful, come up with your own and give it a shot.

No matter how you feel about creating little goals, one easy strategy for increasing or improving nutrition is to create a culture within your family of cooking and eating at home or packing food to go. Food prepared at home tends to be lower in sodium, higher in nutrients, and lower in added sugars. When your child eats meals prepared at home, they likely won't have as much exposure to hyperpalatable foods and will have a lot more exposure to normal foods. This cuts out a lot of the competition between hyperpalatable and normal foods. A potato chip will always catch my attention. A meatball? Not so much. But if spaghetti, meatballs, and broccoli are sitting in front of me and the potato chip is not, the normal food will get my attention. The more normal foods kids have access to, the more their tastes can stay in line with normal food. Taste bud cells die and regenerate quickly (about 10 percent each day) and we can learn to like foods at a less sweet or salty level over the course of about two weeks.

Cooking and eating at home may be a luxury for some families, though it can also save a lot of money. It takes time and coordination. It takes energy and planning. Parents juggling multiple jobs, neurodivergent parents, parents going through stressful situations, and parents without social support may have a hard time planning meals at home. Cooking at home doesn't mean that you have to start making everything from scratch to add in more fruits and veggies. It just means that you have the option to add those fruits and veggies in if you want to.

When you're cooking at home, you can also add in some "extras" in a way that adds nutrients. We usually have some homemade muffins around the house—it's one of the few things we routinely bake—and because we make them ourselves, it's easy to include some add-ins. My muffin recipes usually have some fruit or veggies in them, almost always chocolate chips, and sometimes some seeds or nuts (hemp hearts pack a big protein punch, and chia seeds are loaded with fiber). I'm always looking for ways to add variety, so sometimes I'll grind up a bunch of seeds or nuts in the food processor to make a flour. Then I'll keep the nut/seed flour in the fridge and use it to substitute some of the regular flour when I'm making muffins. I'll also add hemp seeds to oatmeal when I'm cooking a pot of it, add in some shredded carrots to our tuna salad, or soak my french toast sticks in the egg batter for longer to make them high-protein french toast sticks.

Cooking at home also doesn't mean you need to use only the freshest ingredients. I'm still surprised when people talk about frozen veggies and fruit as a compromise, claiming they aren't as nutrient-dense as the fresh version. It's simply not true. Frozen fruits and vegetables are great, full stop. If they make your life easier, use them. They have a different texture than fresh, as well, so your child may enjoy them (or not)—it's another option to try.

Canned foods are also helpful. They also have a different texture and can be easy to store. They often have added sodium and sugar, and sometimes have slightly fewer nutrients, which is why they get a bad rap sometimes, but they are still veggies, and they are still very nutritious. You can rinse them off to decrease added sodium and sugar. Personally, I am exclusively a canned beans person. Every time I decide I'm going to be the person that cooks my own beans, I just am not. The dry beans sit there. Forever. Whispering things like, "When are you going to make us?" "Why haven't you made us yet?" "Why are you using those canned beans instead of us?" After years of listening to whispering dried beans, I finally embraced who I am and stopped buying them. There are other convenience foods that are essential for many of us: bread, sauces, frozen meals, and pre-chopped or -washed foods. These are all good options.

People often want to know what to look for in convenience foods. My answer: If you're in a store making decisions, after you consider what is affordable to you and what your child will actually eat, look for the lowest-sodium or lowest-sugar version, the version that looks the least exciting (boring packaging and no characters), and the version that looks and tastes the most like what you would make at home. After that, you might have the preference to look for the version that has the fewest additives in it.

No matter what kinds of fruits or veggies you buy, I always warn parents about the risks of "sneaking" veggies, fruits, or other ingredients you want your kid to eat more of into foods, especially with picky eaters. Some families can pull this off without their child detecting it, but I've heard enough stories from the parents of picky eaters (or from grown-up picky eaters) to know that often in the end, the picky eater discovers the "hidden" veggies, fruits, or other foods. Then you risk them not eating that food or anything that looks like it for a while. The pickier the eater, the more likely they are to discover little differences that would come from changing ingredients. I often cook things that have veggies, seeds, or oil added in—it's part of my "recipe," but I'll always tell the kids what is in it if they ask. I may put the dish together in front of them or ask them to help me add the ingredients to a recipe we're going to eat together so that they know what's in there.

One day, I was making tacos for my family, and I wanted to use up some mushrooms that were on their way out. One of my kids and I are still learning to like them, but I figured if I chopped them up small enough, it would mix with the taco filling and be fine for us. I wasn't trying to sneak them in, I was trying to use up the ingredient, but it came off looking like I was trying to trick him into eating mushrooms. "Did you put *mushrooms* in this?" he asked. The look of betrayal on his face still haunts me. For the next few months, every time we had tacos, he looked at them suspiciously and asked me if they had mushrooms. This is the exact reason I generally steer clear of sneaking foods into recipes.

On the days when you do decide to eat out, consider ordering a version of a dish that your child will like from the adult menu, which often offers more variety. It also usually doesn't include a drink (which I am convinced—even though I have no hard evidence—is a way to train kids to feel like they need a drink with their meal so that they will buy drinks when they become adults). Plus, adult meals don't come with toys. For years, before my kids could read the menu for themselves and learned there was a kids' menu, we got them spaghetti and broccoli off the adult menu (if we were at a place that did spaghetti and broccoli) and split the meal between them.

THE FIVE QUESTIONS FOR FOOD HEADLINES

Even with knowledge of the six tiers, it's easy to get sidetracked by food and nutrient-related headlines or clean eating content. When the findings of new studies are released, they inevitably get picked up and turned into alarmist clickbait by the media and health content creators. I do what I can to avoid exposure to this kind of anxiety-inducing content, but plenty of alarmist health news still gets to me. When it does, I have to figure out how to interpret the information. Do I ignore it? Do I take it seriously? Here is the process I use to decide.

Step 1: Pause—When I see a health headline, I stop and take a deep breath. During this pause, I don't believe or disbelieve what I've read, I don't comment on it or like it, and I don't share the content.

Step 2: Source—The next thing I do is research the source of the information. Before I consider incorporating a new piece of health information into the way I feed my family, I want to be sure the source is trusted, has followed proper research protocol, and is being kept accountable (by a credentialing board or similar). Having a large social media following unfortunately isn't a good measure of whether someone is a reliable source of information. Part of this step includes finding the original source of the information, because sometimes in the long game of telephone, the original message from the source has gotten mangled (this is almost always true of people "reporting" about research). I also ask myself whether this source might financially benefit if I buy into their headline. If a lawyer is providing information about blood sugar or a health influencer who sells their own protein powder is educating about lead in protein powders, I'm going to be skeptical.

Step 3: Verify—Then I'll take a minute to investigate whether the information sources I already trust have provided information on the topic and if they came to the same conclusion. When I verify information, I always check multiple sources that aren't on social media (an AI response doesn't count). Keep in mind that sources appearing to be "trustworthy" on the surface, even people with credentials, may still be misrepresenting the research (perhaps inadvertently), or using outdated conclusions because they haven't kept up with the latest research on a topic. So steer clear of information provided by sources without relevant experience or training, especially those quoting and screenshotting AI conversations and summaries—AI is often wrong when it comes to food and nutrition information, and someone with in-depth knowledge won't use an AI summary as a source. Stay a bit skeptical of everyone.

Once you establish that you do (even if a bit skeptically) trust a source, use the following five questions to help you decide whether health-related content deserves your attention and action. These questions will keep you from wasting energy on information that isn't serving you.

1. *Is the content nuanced and free from sensationalism?* "Candy is slowly poisoning all children" is a statement that is sensational without any nuance. "When children eat large amounts of candy, it spikes their blood sugar, but when a small amount of candy is eaten with a balanced meal, it does not" is a statement that is nuanced and free from sensationalism.
2. *Does my child eat a lot of the food in question?* If you see a headline that says LEAD FOUND IN TOP 50 CHOCOLATE BRANDS but your child eats only a few chocolate chips once a week, the answer to this question is *no*, and you can feel free to disregard the headline.

3. *Can I swap in a different food my child will eat for the ingredient in question without decreasing their nutrition and variety?* Let's say, for example, the content is about heavy metals in sweet potatoes, and you are considering removing sweet potatoes from your child's diet as a result. However, your child is unwilling to eat any other foods that are high in vitamin A, so your answer to this question is *no*. A vitamin A deficiency is likely much more dangerous than whatever the headline said is wrong with the sweet potato.
4. *Do I have the time, money, or energy to avoid the ingredient in question?* If you would need to cut other important things from your spending or time to swap to the "better for you" foods, then the answer is *no*.
5. *Is my child already doing okay when it comes to the "top tiers"?* If your child isn't eating enough protein or fiber, or getting the vitamins and minerals they need, then the answer is *no* (the only exception is if the information makes it into one of the top tiers like being a source of heavy metal poisoning or food recalls). If you will have to take time, mental energy, or finances away from one of the top tiers to address this headline, the answer is *no*.

If your answer to *any* one of these questions is *no*, move on. This latest piece of food news is not worth paying attention to. Good-quality information is not usually sensational, and it should provide details and nuance. With that said, usually the sensational food information in the media has a grain of truth to it. For example, I saw a sensational video this year created by someone who was calling baby carrots "toxic" because they are washed in "chlorine." Now, baby carrots *can* be washed in a diluted chlorinated wash. But after the diluted chlorinated wash, they are washed with water to remove the chlorine—it's not optional; there are regulations requiring a specific washing procedure. This chlorine bath is done to prevent bacteria from growing on carrots, which can make us sick. So, while the sensationalized video made it sound like baby carrots are soaking in little bags of pool water, the reality is that ready-to-eat produce usually goes through a sanitizing wash-and-rinse procedure so that you don't get something nasty like listeria poisoning from eating them. If you hear someone say that an otherwise healthy food is "poisonous" or "toxic," that's a sign that the information is sensational and taken out of context.

Moving on to the other questions. With #2, if your child isn't eating a lot of the food in question, then the risks from this specific food are going to be very low. For #3, the biggest risk from removing foods is that you must replace them, which will risk decreasing the variety and nutrients in your child's diet if there's not a new nutritious replacement that your child will eat. Additionally, it means your child will eat more of another food, increasing their exposure to whatever contaminant or risk is associated with that food. For #4, if you don't have the time, money, or energy to make a change, then you simply cannot make that change, practically speaking. And for #5, if your child doesn't have the big things taken care of, the little things aren't going to make a big difference for their health.

However, if your answer to all of these questions is *yes*, then you might consider serving less of that food to your child.

SUPPLEMENTS

The kids' supplement market has taken on a life of its own. Parents constantly ask me which pills, powders, shakes, gummies, vitamin drops, minerals, and other nutrients they should buy for their child. Supplements are a tool. There are three reasons for supplementation: 1) deficiency prevention, 2) treating deficiency, 3) therapeutic use for specific health conditions. We'll talk about deficiency prevention here, and then deficiency treatment and therapeutic use in chapter 14.

If your child is getting enough of the recommended nutrients from their diet, there is no need for them to take supplements. However, we know from the data that a significant number of children in the US are *not* getting all the nutrients they need. You can guess whether your child might benefit from taking a supplement either by comparing what they eat with the Health Impact Tiers recommendations, tracking the nutrients they are getting from dietary sources and comparing that with the recommended intakes, or by testing their nutrient levels through laboratory tests such as blood work.

DEFICIENCY PREVENTION

If your child is not getting adequate nutrition from their diet, a supplement may be able to fill in the gap between what they eat and what they need to prevent a deficiency. Most children's multivitamins are used for this purpose. They usually don't contain a full day's worth of nutrients, but they are meant to provide a variety of nutrients, assuming you'll be providing the rest via diet. There is still risk, however, that taking a multivitamin may bump your child's intake of certain nutrients above the healthy, recommended range. Additionally, some children should not take multivitamins given other conditions that they have. This is why it's important to talk to your child's healthcare provider before starting them on a multivitamin. If your healthcare provider gives you the green light, then the risk of harm from taking a children's multivitamin is low.

I have observed that sometimes when stressed parents give their child a multivitamin, they feel less worried, which allows them to relax more at mealtimes, which in turn allows their child to relax more at mealtimes, which enables the child to eat more variety at mealtimes. If that's the case for you, then go for it. I don't hold a strong position on using or not using multivitamins with kids if parents have checked with their child's healthcare provider that they don't have ingredients that could be dangerous for their child. (One exception: I do have a strong position against supplement companies that deceptively lead parents to believe their once-daily vitamin will fix their child's emotional outbursts or whatever the complaint is. A simple multivitamin will not solve your child's deficiencies or behavioral challenges.)

A more accurate way to supplement, however, is by giving your child only the nutrients they are not eating enough of. My kids don't eat enough vitamin D, so I give them a vitamin D supplement. They also don't eat fish often enough to meet their omega-3 fatty acid needs, so I give them a supplement for that, too. They eat enough vitamin C, however, so I don't supplement vitamin C. Here's what I recommend for deficiency prevention if you are worried about it and are wondering about whether a supplement might be useful for your child:

1. Track what your child eats for three to seven days to find out how many nutrients they are getting, and compare that to the recommended intakes.
2. If there is a gap between what your child eats and the recommendations, contact your child's healthcare provider to let them know which supplements you are considering and to find out if supplements may be harmful for your child.
3. Don't over-supplement—more is not always better (or safe) when it comes to supplements.

POWDERS AND POTIONS

The supplement industry is not regulated in the same way the pharmaceutical industry is. For example, in most cases, the Food and Drug Administration (FDA) is not authorized to test the effectiveness or safety of supplements before they are put on the market, and the FDA has said they do not have the resources to test all supplements to determine their safety. While supplement companies are supposed to ensure their products are safe and properly labeled, that doesn't always happen, and for the most part, no one is checking up on them. The exception is companies who decide to have their product *third-party tested.* That means another company checks their formulas to ensure quality and ingredients. I highly recommend purchasing only products that are third-party tested.

Supplements are not without value—some are evidence-based and become an important part of a person's healthcare. But be aware of who is recommending them to you and what their motives might be. The supplement industry is extremely lucrative. As a registered dietitian, I have access to a professional-grade supplement dispensary. I can get clinician pricing, and if I wanted to, I could sell supplements to others at a *very large* markup (though I don't choose to do that). Many influencers and practitioners sell supplements to their followers as a source of income, however. So beware of whose advice on supplements you are taking and whether they are making a profit on those recommendations. Make sure you vet the person selling the supplements using the steps above before considering purchasing supplements from someone online—and unless they can explain the nuances of when someone should and shouldn't take them, find a different source to purchase from.

Learning to eat what nourishes us is a lifelong endeavor. The nutrients that our kids need will change as they age and grow, and it helps to acknowledge that nourishing our kids is a long-haul job that comes with a lot of ups and downs. If, after reading this section, you recognize that you are hitting only the top two tiers of child feeding, accept that this is the best you can do for now. Your best is best, and you're allowed to feel good about nailing tier 1 (Living) and tier 2 (Growing). You'll be able to do more in the future, so when you are able, add on some tier 3 (Thriving) elements to your child's diet. That will feel good, too. For now, work within what's realistic for your family, and don't let all the food noise distract you from focusing on what you know will be best for your child.

PART II

A SIX-STEP PLAN FOR NAVIGATING FOOD DILEMMAS

6

NAVIGATING REAL-LIFE DILEMMAS WITH CONFIDENCE

"My stepdaughter has been diagnosed with obesity, and I can see her gaining weight. I don't want to draw any attention to her size. I'm also watching her use food to numb and cope with all her stresses. Everyone is saying to leave her alone and not worry about it, which I get, but what's happening is not healthy for her. I feel like we're letting her down by doing nothing."

"My son is extremely picky and only eats seven foods. He's anemic now. We never pressure him, and we've been exposing him to foods for his whole life, but he never tries a new food."

"My son is newly type 1 diabetic. Sometimes I really need him to eat or he can't have something because of his insulin, so I have to force him to eat something or restrict him. I always feel like I'm ruining his relationship with food."

While I stand by the "best" practices in part 1 of this book, there will be times when you simply cannot follow them. These are the feeding dilemmas that we'll discuss throughout part 2. They include relationships with relatives and friends, eating challenges—from starting solid foods to chaos at mealtimes, then picky eating and extreme picky eating / ARFID, challenges with your child's relationship with sweets, their body, and eating disorders, and therapeutic diets and health conditions. Your particular feeding struggle, whatever it may be, may make these practices impossible. But even in these difficult moments, there are steps you can take to minimize the risk of whatever "less-than-ideal" feeding approach you must take. These steps won't "fix" a specific eating challenge, but they will help you understand your options, minimize harm, make choices intentionally, and do what makes the most sense for your family. Even in the moment of a dilemma, you are in charge. And that alone can give you courage.

A SIX-STEP PLAN FOR NAVIGATING FOOD DILEMMAS

The following six-step framework can be used to navigate just about any tricky feeding dilemma that you encounter with your kids.

First, we need to acknowledge that our assumptions, emotions, and imaginations can get in the way of us finding the right solution for a situation. We might be imagining the worst-case scenario or assume we're failing as parents. Stories like these usually drain our motivation and creativity. So, in step 1, we "separate fact from fiction" and take on a calmer and more rational, hopeful perspective.

In step 2, we have to make a tough choice about what we will prioritize in our situation. It's easy to get stuck trying to figure out what to do when we are trying to make everyone happy or solve *all* the problems. That's not possible when it comes to dilemmas. So no matter how uncomfortable, we pick the priority.

Step 3 is to brainstorm strategies to support your priority. You will note all your ideas, whether they are realistic or ridiculous, and in this case, even ideas you think are bad. When it comes to dilemmas, there are no easy solutions, and we have to think outside the box. You will also note the pros and cons of each of the strategies that you come up with, and then you add a twist—you use words like *may* and *might*—because these words remind you that you don't know what will happen, and this helps you be more willing to accept unconventional strategies to move forward.

Step 4 includes acknowledging that any strategy you try will come with risks, especially because dilemmas mean you won't be able to use all the best practices you might wish you could. Still, even if you need to use a riskier strategy, that doesn't mean the outcome is out of your control. You will have many opportunities to minimize the risks of whatever approach you choose. This is called a *risk reduction approach*.

Once you decide on your approach, it's time for step 5: taking on the mind of a scientist and thinking of these strategies as an experiment. Because dilemmas are so complicated, we don't really know what will happen when we try a specific strategy. It may be a complete flop, or it may be great. We need to go in with the understanding that we will try something and then watch and see how it goes.

Finally, in step 6, we celebrate and continue experimenting. Taking a moment to celebrate going through the process and starting an experiment gives you a chance to feel successful—as you should! Navigating dilemmas can feel like a thankless task, so we have to give ourselves positive feedback—we went through the hard work of starting an experiment. Great job! And then we get right back to work, observing our outcomes and deciding whether we want to keep going in that direction or if we need to make changes and try something else.

Step 1: Separate fact from fiction.

Step 2: Pick the priority.

Step 3: Brainstorm—with a twist.

Step 4: Take a risk reduction approach.

Step 5: Think like a scientist and start an experiment.

Step 6: Celebrate your wins, then continue to tweak your experiment.

In this chapter, I will walk you through how each of these six steps works by using one family's dilemma as a case study. But keep in mind that the six steps can be applied to any of the tricky feeding situations that I discuss in the chapters throughout part 2. If your family is facing a particular feeding dilemma at this moment, I encourage you to grab pen and paper (or your laptop) and jot down your own responses, using this framework to problem-solve.

Annie's Family's Story

The parents of a one-year-old girl named Annie prefer to reduce her exposure to sweets as much as possible during toddlerhood. However, Grandma and Grandpa babysit for Annie regularly. They love spoiling their granddaughter and they give her many sweets throughout the day whenever they babysit for her, despite knowing her parents want to limit her sweets as a young toddler. Grandma and Grandpa watch Annie for free, and Annie's parents would otherwise struggle to pay for childcare, so they are reluctant to speak up and object about this for fear of creating conflict or seeming ungrateful.

STEP 1: SEPARATE FACT FROM FICTION

The first step involves establishing the facts of the situation with as little emotional spin as possible. When you are in the middle of a tricky feeding situation, sometimes it's hard to figure out how big a problem you are dealing with and what is truly at risk. This step will help put the problem into perspective and take some of the emotional power out of it.

Consider the following two questions, and jot down your immediate responses:

- What is the dilemma?
- What is your desired outcome?

Here is what Annie's parents wrote down in response:

The dilemma: *We don't want our toddler to have sweets, but we love the grandparents, need free childcare, and don't want to seem ungrateful for the help.*

The desired outcome: *Annie won't be given sweets at Grandma and Grandpa's, we'll continue to have a good relationship with the grandparents, and the grandparents will continue to provide free childcare.*

Next, we're going to separate the facts we've just established from the fictional "story" we're telling ourselves to the side. It can be tricky to figure out the best course of action when we're wrapped up in the "story" that we're telling ourselves. You already wrote down the facts. Now you're going to write down the "story," which includes things like what you worry might happen in the future, and the stories you are telling yourself about why people are doing what they are doing. Whether the story is true or not doesn't matter. It's just important to get it out of your head and down on the page.

Ask yourself the following questions, and jot down your responses:

- What are you afraid will happen in the future if this situation continues?
- What stories are you telling yourself?

Here is what Annie's parents wrote down in response.

Their fears:

- *Annie will get sick more often from eating too much sugar.*
- *She'll be less willing to eat fruits, vegetables, and non-sweet foods.*
- *She'll demand lots of sweets.*
- *If we say something, there will be a huge break in the relationship with grandparents, who will be offended.*
- *Grandparents will stop providing childcare.*
- *One of us might lose a job.*
- *We might experience financial difficulties.*

The stories they were telling themselves:

- *Grandparents don't care about Annie's health.*
- *Grandparents don't respect us as parents, so they won't follow our wishes.*
- *Annie will always be obsessed with sweets because of this.*

STEP 2: PICK THE PRIORITY

Now it's time to decide what's most important to you. You may be juggling multiple goals, but you need to choose one to focus on. Figure out which is the most pressing by writing down all your goals. If someone's livelihood or immediate physical or mental health is at risk, that likely carries the most weight. All your goals are important, but only one can be the top priority for this step. As you are writing, think past the immediate situation to what you really want. For example, you won't see "Reduce sugar" on this family's goal list. Their daughter's health is the goal, not reducing sugar.

This is where the dilemma hits hard, because you will likely have to put something else that feels important a little lower on the list. Your family will have unique priorities. There is no wrong answer here. Grab your pencil and paper, or laptop, and:

- Make a list of goals.
- Prioritize the goals and choose the number one problem to address.

Annie's family's goals:

- *Top priority: Maintain good family relationships.*
- *Keep jobs.*
- *Don't experience financial hardship.*
- *Help Annie be healthy.*
- *Help Annie eat a wide variety of foods.*

For this family, sustaining strong relationships with Grandma and Grandpa is of the utmost importance. These bonds are important to Mom and Dad, and the fact that the grandparents provide childcare is also meaningful. Preserving that arrangement is crucial to both parents keeping their jobs and saving on the high costs of day care or a babysitter. While the parents absolutely want to keep their child healthy and eating a wide variety of foods—the "healthy" that is sacrificed with some additional sweets is less vital. Having Annie eat a wide variety of foods, while ideal, is not what's most important to the family overall.

STEP 3: BRAINSTORM—WITH A TWIST

It's time to take action. Even deciding *not* to take action is an action. Brainstorm your various options and write them down as a list, making sure not to edit out things that on the surface seem like a bad idea. This is curiosity in action. Leaving out possibilities you think are "not ideal" or "a compromise" during a brainstorm is often where parents get stuck and run out of choices or end up using strategies that aren't a good fit. Remember, there's no guarantee of how *your* child will react to a strategy—no matter how popular or unpopular it is. Don't limit yourself at this step.

You can come up with your own list of actions, and keep in mind that the rest of part 2 will offer additional actions and strategies that you might add to your list for various specific dilemmas.

Annie's family's possible actions:

- *Say nothing to grandparents and let things continue as they are.*
- *Ask grandparents to stop giving sweets completely.*
- *Ask grandparents to partially stop giving sweets.*
- *Find new childcare arrangement.*

Next, we're going to evaluate our possible actions by creating a pros-and-cons list. The "twist" is that we don't know what will happen, right? We know from the research that not all actions have the same outcomes for every child. Use words like *may*, *might*, *could*, *possibly*, and *maybe* in your pros-and-cons list. Hopefully, this reminds you that nothing is for certain.

Think through each of the actions that you have noted, and list what you imagine could go wrong or right. In the rest of the chapters of part 2, I'll be giving some examples of why actions might work for certain kids and not for others.

STEP 4: TAKE A RISK REDUCTION APPROACH

Let's imagine a parent telling this story: "It was a snow day, so the kids were home. I also had several important work meetings and deadlines that I couldn't miss, so I had them watch TV the entire day. I picked lots of nature documentaries since they feel more calming, and that way, we'd have something to talk about later. I

ACTION	POSSIBLE PROS	POSSIBLE CONS
Say nothing to grandparents and let things continue as they are	Probably will maintain good family relationships Probably free childcare continues	Parents may resent grandparents Child may develop strong preference for sweets Child may not consume enough nutrient-dense foods
Ask grandparents to stop giving sweets completely	Child may eat fewer sweets Parents may be less worried about child Grandparents may be happy to stop	Grandparents may be offended There may be relationship fallout Free childcare may be jeopardized Grandparents may not change anything There may be mutual resentment between the parents and grandparents Financial hardship may occur
Ask grandparents to partially stop	Child may eat fewer sweets Parents may be less worried about child Grandparents may be willing to make partial change	Grandparents may be offended There may be relationship fallout Free childcare may be jeopardized Grandparents may not change anything Parents may still resent grandparents Financial hardship may occur Child may develop preference for sweets
Find a new childcare arrangement	Child may eat fewer sweets Parents may be less worried about child's health	Financial hardship likely Relationship fallout likely

also chose some shows that included physical activities in hopes that they'd get off the couch and move around."

A public health researcher would refer to what this parent did as a *risk reduction approach*. Risk reduction is an evidence-based approach used in many fields, and it's an excellent tool for parents to use when it comes to handling child feeding dilemmas. Risk reduction is about using a strategy to make an activity less risky. Life is full of risks, and we are constantly employing strategies as parents to mitigate these risks for our children. We make our kids wear helmets, we put child locks on cabinets with cleaning supplies, we put squirmy toddlers in a five-point harness in the car. The parent above knew it wasn't great for their children to watch TV the *whole* day and that it came with some risks or drawbacks, but given the situation, it was the solution they decided was best. So the parent used some risk reduction strategies, including choosing shows that were educational and soothing for their kids, shows that could lead to some family conversations later, and shows that could potentially lead to the kids moving around. There's a good chance the kids may have no ill effects from this day—or, if they have some, it's likely they will have less.

The "best practices" or "methods" that professionals and specialists recommend are often the practices that have the least risk of harm to the most people. Just for fun, let's pick one of the most emotionally charged hot-button topics in child feeding: breastfeeding versus formula feeding. I can easily recommend breastfeeding because it's a practice that runs the least risk of harm to the most people. Breastfeeding has been studied at length, and as a result, it's considered the best practice in infant feeding. It's actually a collection of practices, though—there's the social connection, the physical connection, the teaching of latching or sucking, and more. It also prevents some unhelpful things from happening. For example, you can't mistakenly mix the wrong amount of water into breast milk, and breast milk is nutritionally sound on its own. It's also hard to force-feed a breastfed baby compared with a bottle-fed baby, which makes it easier to respect their fullness cues. Finally, it's trickier to be emotionally disconnected with breastfeeding, because there is mandatory skin-to-skin contact and the baby is right in front of your face. It's a bunch of strategies bundled together and called the "breastfeeding" method.

When a "best practice" isn't the best choice for a family, however, that family may need to take a risk reduction approach. So let's imagine what a risk reduction approach might look like for a family for whom breastfeeding is not possible, and thus not a best practice. If the "ideal" scenario is a mother exclusively breastfeeding and emotionally connecting with her infant and both of them thriving, the worst-case scenario is a baby failing to thrive because they weren't fed sufficiently and/or were only fed via propping a bottle up into the baby's mouth so that no one needed to sit there and feed them and they didn't get enough human nurturing.

Risk reduction can be thought of as a ladder, with the bottom rung having the most risk of harm and the top having the least risk. The list below is one portion of the infant feeding ladder—there are of course other more detailed rungs that I didn't include, but this can give you an idea of what a ladder looks like up close:

1. Insufficient feeding that leads to malnutrition
2. Sufficient formula or breast milk, even if it's a bad digestive fit for the baby, with bottle propping
3. Sufficient formula or breast milk that's a good digestive fit, and a caregiver who emotionally engages with the infant but force-feeds
4. Sufficient formula or breast milk and an emotionally available caregiver who force-feeds less
5. A mix of formula and breast milk with an emotionally available caregiver who honors hunger cues

The ladder continues with more rungs that reduce more risks. But at some point, many babies will stop experiencing any harms or risks altogether, even if the person isn't practicing the full "ideal" scenario. For example, if a family is giving their baby "sufficient formula or breast milk from an emotionally available caregiver who force-feeds *less*," many babies won't be experiencing any risk of harm at all. Some babies may need to be force-fed *sometimes* due to a medical condition, but they will still experience the good nutrition and emotional nurturing that can protect them from the risks of force-feeding, because they are force-fed *less*, only when it's essential, instead of it being the norm for feeding the child.

A risk reduction approach can help you maintain a healthier perspective, because you'll be able to see that there are a lot of good things you are already doing. It also gives you options to reduce your child's risks and find the path that is best for them, and to see that there's a good chance you don't have to be on the top rung to avoid harm befalling your child or someone else.

Let's return to the story of Annie and the sweets. For this step in the dilemma navigation process, you're going to make another list. Ask yourself: *How can I reduce the risk of the "cons" with each of the actions I am considering?* Then list the ways in which you can take a risk reduction approach to that action. Annie's parents are considering asking the grandparents to offer fewer sweets, and taking a risk reduction approach in this situation would involve asking this of the grandparents, followed by taking some or all of the following risk reduction actions.

Possible risk reduction actions:

- Tell the grandparents how much we love them, want Annie to have a good relationship with them, and how grateful we are for their help raising Annie.
- Take a respectful approach to bringing up this touchy subject with the grandparents, and show them that we understand their perspective by saying something like, "We

know you love to spoil her—you're her grandparents! And we know it's important for her to have treats sometimes." This will help them know we are on their side and will help smooth a sticky conversation, which will ideally lead to more flexibility on their part.

- Make things easy for the grandparents. If we provide them with all the snacks they will need for Annie throughout the day or the flexibility they need, it will be easier for them to make a change and thus lessen their potential frustration with our request.
- Offer to meet the grandparents halfway and still allow them to give Annie some sweets (but not as many as they were giving her before). If there is too much change requested, it might be too hard for them to even think of changing, so compromising on something that is a smaller change may be more motivating.

Annie's parents decide to ask the grandparents to stop serving sweets to her daily and to instead limit them to an agreed-upon number. They know that it's a best practice to delay the introduction of sweets to toddlers, but they also know it's not the best or most practical option for their situation. By taking this risk reduction approach, some of the risks are still possible for their child, but negative consequences are reduced compared with letting the grandparents continue their current practices. Because maintaining the relationship is their highest priority, they decide to do everything possible to make this a positive and easy change for the grandparents.

STEP 5: THINK LIKE A SCIENTIST AND START AN EXPERIMENT

Now it's time to find out how the action you choose will work in your family by thinking like a scientist and putting your curiosity into full gear. This is an "experiment," because you can change course at any time. You are not committing to it forever, although allowing an action some time to take effect is often a good idea. There is no "right" or "best" action here, because you're navigating a dilemma.

You have chosen your action, and now it's time to start your risk reduction plan. In the early days of your experiment, you can pay special attention to what happens, and what changes, after you start. Take notes if you're a note-taking kind of person. Here is what Annie's family did once they put their risk reduction plan into action:

> *Annie's mother called Annie's grandmother during a time when she knew the grandmother would be in a good mood.*
>
> **Mom:** "Hey, Mom. Annie's doctor has recommended she not eat sweets at this age so that she still has room in her tummy for the nutrients she needs."
>
> **Grandma:** "That's ridiculous. You're depriving her."
>
> **Mom:** "Annie loves you so much, she adores you, and we want to make sure she has a good relationship with you. We're also so grateful for the time you spend with her and watching her. I know how much you love to give her sweets. We're okay with that; we'd like to keep it to three small sweets a week, though. She also has these other snacks that she's obsessed with and are a huge treat for her even though they aren't sweets. We can stop serving them at home so that she only has them at your house. She'll still have all the treats with you. We'll keep you stocked."
>
> **Grandma:** "Three times a week isn't enough. She should have a sweet every day."
>
> **Mom:** "All right, we can work with that. She can have one small sweet each day. Can we try it for three weeks and see how it goes? We can always change back to the way it was if it's not going well."
>
> **Grandma:** "Okay, fine. I can't wait to kiss those cute little cheeks of hers on Monday!"

STEP 6: CELEBRATE YOUR WINS, THEN CONTINUE TO TWEAK YOUR EXPERIMENT

You prepared, you made a decision, you're courageously running an experiment and gathering data. You are owning your role as an intentional parent. The truth is, this process never ends. Annie's parents will likely continue to have conversations with the grandparents about sugar or some other feeding challenge, depending on how everyone changes over time. Still, every time you implement a change, you should celebrate that you did it. It's not about the outcome but the fact that you're making decisions, going through the process, and seeing small glimmers of success. That's not easy, and it deserves acknowledgment!

Keep in mind, the celebration is not the end. Once you've given yourself a moment to take in your success, you should get back to being curious and paying attention to your experiment and its outcomes. You might find that everything is going well and doesn't need much adjustment. Or you might find that you aren't seeing any benefits and that your current strategy isn't working. Keep an open mind. It's better to recognize any hiccups early and then tweak your experiment, or set up a new one. This is good data! Learning that a strategy doesn't work doesn't make you a bad parent or someone ruining their kids; it makes you a real parent. Now it's time to look for a strategy that *will* work.

So, did the experiment with Annie's grandparents work? Let's return to it:

Annie's parents watch how things are going with the grandparents.

The grandparents have been keeping up their end of the bargain, and their daughter has been having only one small sweet a day, along with plenty of her favorite snacks brought from home. The parents give Grandma a call, thank her for what she's doing, and ask how things are going and if they can try it for another month. Grandma grumbles a bit, but also says it's going fine and that she's willing to keep doing only one sweet a day for another month. Annie also continues to eat a variety of foods at home.

Annie's parents feel good that Grandma is on board for the next month, and they accomplished their number one priority of maintaining a good relationship. They feel confident that they navigated a tricky situation and have started their first experiment. They also know that neither grandparent really approves and both make snide comments any chance they get even though they're going along with it. The parents are disappointed that they won't be able to reduce sweets as much as they wanted and that they don't have the full support of the grandparents. They know that this is part of parenting, though, and they can still do so many things to help their child be healthy and learn to like a variety of foods.

Overall, this experiment is working out. For the time being, Annie's parents stick with it. But they intend to keep an eye on the comments to be sure nothing is being said about sweets in front of Annie. For now, no major changes are needed, but the observation continues.

7

FEEDING DISAGREEMENTS

When Family Members, Loved Ones, and Friends Feed Differently

"My partner insists on making my child finish their plate."

"My mother won't stop telling my six-year-old daughter to 'take it easy if you want to keep your figure.'"

"My child is an extreme picky eater, and she just can't eat food that other people make. My friend was so offended when we brought a special meal for my daughter."

The example in the previous chapter, about Annie and her grandparents, dealt with extended family members who pile on the sweets or disapprove of parents' approach to hyperpalatable foods, but there are so many ways in which your loved ones' approach to feeding can affect your child. This is good news, in this regard, if your child has many people who care about them. That's a gift! But when there are many different people who feed them, some of those people may approach eating from a different perspective, or with different preferences, convictions, and beliefs, than you do. Being on the same page with those who routinely feed your child—including family members, friends, and caregivers—can be helpful for kids. But sometimes this is easier said than done. Disagreements about feeding between two parents, or parents and grandparents and other relatives, are common, so common that the food dilemma framework in chapter 6 used an example of this type of disagreement. Sometimes these dilemmas are so intense that they may jeopardize the quality of the relationships. Picking which battles to prioritize can be tricky for families.

Sofia and Lydia

Sofia (age ten), Lydia (age eight), and their parents often have dinner with their extended family on the weekends. Some relatives openly discuss their weight-loss diets, and several of them, including Grandma, have recently started to comment on Sofia's weight and body size. This type of talk has always been part of family gatherings, but Sofia recently told her parents she should go on a diet to lose weight.

Sofia and Lydia's parents have worked hard to foster a positive perspective on bodies in their home. They taught the girls that it's not okay to talk about other people's bodies without their permission. They have also been careful not to say negative things about their own bodies or weigh themselves in front of the kids. They have tried giving Grandma and all their relatives hints that they shouldn't discuss diets around the kids, but they have been ignored. Now that Sofia says she wants to go on a diet, her parents know it's urgent to intervene.

WHAT'S GOING ON?

Food and feeding—especially feeding kids—are emotionally charged topics. Food touches our health, values, politics, traditions, parenting, culture, connection to other people, and more. We were all fed, so we have ingrained practices that feel right to us. If we disagree with someone else's food practices and communicate this disagreement, they may feel that we are saying their way is wrong. Our relationships with our bodies and our experiences with diet culture and health are also deeply personal, emotional, and individualized. Some cultures and people take a more collectivist perspective, where the well-being of the group is prioritized over an individual's needs. This may contribute to the adults in a child's life all wanting to use different feeding practices. On top of it all, your child comes to the table with their own temperament, feelings, and needs.

START WITH THE BASICS

PICK YOUR BATTLES

Since feeding kids can be emotionally loaded, any conversations or practices related to food and your child can feel high stakes. That doesn't mean that they actually *are* all high stakes, however. You have to decide how important the issue at the heart of your food disagreement is to you. Some actions, like Lydia and Sofia's family discussing their weight or weight shaming, are objectively high risk across the board. Force-feeding and neglecting tier 1 nutrition needs also fall into that category. Others may be high stakes for you (based on your values) or your child (based on their needs), such as a decision to be vegetarian, following a religious diet, a child's picky eating tendencies, your desire to handle restriction differently based on personal experience of restriction, or your child's strong desire for independence.

Situations with family and friends can be tricky to navigate, but remember that *you* are your child's advocate. Your child will be depending on you to help them work through relationship dynamics, family traditions, and community and personal needs. There will probably be times where it makes sense to be the "bad guy" and confront or hold boundaries with family and friends, and other times where you can just roll your eyes (to yourself) and let it go.

If you've decided a situation is important enough to address, start by trying some basic strategies that usually don't come with a lot of risk.

When facing this issue, we would all benefit from embracing kindness and patience as two of our virtues. You'll need to exercise kindness and patience toward yourself, but also toward anyone else involved in feeding your child. They will never do it "perfectly," and they will be bringing their own experiences and relationship with food to the task as well. There may be times when the person who is charged with feeding your kids will not be willing to change their practices to match yours, and you won't be able to lessen your child's exposure to them. In cases like these, you'll need to stay grounded and keep any anger or frustration at bay as you decide how to navigate the issue. Remember, in most circumstances, everyone is doing what they think is best. Everyone wants your child to be healthy and happy. When you keep that in mind, it's easier to be more generous and tolerant, whether you decide to let this one go or address it head-on.

COMMUNICATE

There's no way around this one. You're going to have to share your thoughts with the person or people involved in feeding your child if you want them to change their behavior. It may not be easy, but there are ways to make it eas*ier*. To start, communicate your desires and boundaries ahead of time. If you wait until you're in the moment of disagreement, the other person may be caught off guard, and emotions can get ramped up quickly.

Plan to reach out at a time that you know will be convenient for the other person, and use the communication style that *they* (not you!) like best—text, voice/video recording, phone call, email, and so on. Practice what you want to say ahead of time or jot down some notes, and start with something positive like, "We're so excited to see you next week!" or "Thanks so much for inviting us over for dinner!" Then make it clear in your communication that you are giving them the benefit of the doubt and that everyone has the shared goal of helping your child to be as healthy as possible.

No matter how angry or frustrated you are, don't suggest that the person you're talking to has done anything wrong. Let them know the *why* behind the conversation. You might say, "Sofia is starting to have negative thoughts about her body because of what she is hearing at dinners, and we want to help her love her body." Or, "David has extreme picky eating. We're working on it with him, but he needs specific foods right now."

When you bring up your child's needs or changes you want to be made, people can easily get defensive. If you're talking to your parents, they may take personal offense, assuming you think they did it wrong and that's why you're doing it differently. Others might think your comments imply that they are intentionally hurting your child in some way or that they cook poorly. They may try to change the subject or insult you or your parenting. They may do or say something else that makes you want to defend yourself or stand up for your beliefs. Don't get roped into drama or tangents (even on important topics). Often, these tangents make the conversation more emotionally charged and take away from the goal of the talk, which is to ask them to change something for your child's well-being. You can come back to the other issues another time.

If you're speaking with your partner, ask them about their observations, opinions, concerns (or lack of concerns), and their take on the situation. Then listen carefully to their thoughts and observations. Keep an open mind so that you can find common ground.

Finally, no matter who you are talking to, acknowledge their needs and how you are working on meeting them halfway. For example, Sofia and Lydia's mother might say to Grandma, "I know you want to talk about your diet. Can you give me all the updates while she is playing outside with the cousins?" or David's mother might say, "My favorite family dish! I'll eat enough for both of us!" And always close the conversation on a positive note, like thanking this person for their support, or reminding them how much you and your child appreciate having them in your life.

MAKE CHANGE EASY

Since you are the person who is asking for change, do what you can to make that change easy for everyone involved. If the event in question is a family dinner, you might bring food for your child or a dish to share, bring a new game for people to play, or have a list of conversation topics in your head that can engage people quickly. If you want a grandparent to spoil your child with treats less often, they might appreciate a list of other ways they can spoil your child that don't involve food. If there is a way to take some of the burden off the person you are asking to change, it will become easier for them to do what you would like them to do.

TEACH YOUR CHILD TO ADVOCATE FOR THEMSELVES

Depending on your child's age, you can help them learn to respond in appropriate and clear ways by saying things like, "I'm full, and I don't need to finish my plate," "I'm allergic to . . . ," or, simply, "No thank you." If someone around them is talking about their body, your child may be able to say something like "I don't want to talk about this," "I need to go to the bathroom," or simply walk away from the situation.

PROBLEM-SOLVING STRATEGIES TO TRY

The strategies in this section involve compromise and risk reduction, so keep in mind as you consider them that they mean you won't get to do things *exactly* the way you had hoped. However, the goal here is to prioritize and provide your child with the healthiest possible experience. Curiosity is your best friend when thinking about risk reduction. Even if someone approaches feeding your child in a way you disagree with, it may still be okay for your child. Get curious about whether there are elements of the other person's approach that may also be valuable.

AGREE TO SERVE LESS IF THERE'S A "CLEAN PLATE CLUB"

If a friend or family member requires that your child finish their plate, see if you can come to an agreement with the other person on serving smaller portions. If portions are small, a child will be less likely to overeat or eat past the point of fullness, even if they must finish their plate.

MAKE YOUR REQUEST SMALLER

Compromise can come in many forms. If you can't get complete buy-in from another person, they may be willing to agree to a smaller request. For example, if you would rather your child's caregiver delay all sweets but they won't comply, you might be able to get them to agree to delay some sweets. Or let's say you really want your relatives to talk about foods neutrally and without mention of calories around your child. Your relatives, however, are not interested in a complete language overhaul, and you know they will continue to categorize foods as good or bad. You can't take a complete pause from interacting with them at this time, so instead of asking for all of it, maybe you request that they stop talking about calories specifically. They may still call foods good or bad, but there is less risk since they are now talking about one less thing related to diet culture.

Perhaps your partner is very controlling and restrictive with food and your child is beginning to sneak foods, lie about what they ate, and obsessively overeat sweets. You may wonder if your child's reactance is being triggered and, if so, if giving your child more freedom with food would be helpful for them. Rather than advocating for an "open sweets" policy with your partner, however, where your child is allowed to have unlimited sweets whenever they want (which would likely be a bridge too far), it might be helpful to advocate for just one element of structured permission. You might ask your partner if they would be willing to use more warmth and fewer qualifications when speaking to your child about sweets. Or perhaps your family could create a sweets routine where your child knows when the sweets will be available, even if it is not often enough to be fully satisfying to them. Whatever your solution, you may have to start small.

PROVIDE AN ALTERNATIVE

If someone is going to give your child foods that you'd rather they not have, there may be a way for you to provide alternative foods that still make them happy but that get a little bit closer to your goals. This may include lower-sugar cookies, diluted juice, or lower-sodium snacks.

PRACTICE INTERRUPTING, CHANGING THE SUBJECT, OR LEAVING THE AREA

I'm not one to have quick comebacks or good one-liners on the spot, so I need to have a plan ahead of time. There are times, however, when unhelpful conversations come up and I must react then and there. If you need to interrupt conversations that you believe are going to have a negative effect on your child, you might say something simple like, "I need to interrupt here," or "That's a topic for a different time." You can also change the subject or remove yourself or your kids from the conversation by taking a bathroom break or sending the kids outside to play.

PRACTICE AHEAD OF TIME

Your child can always learn new skills—in fact, it's good for them! Help them learn and practice skills, such as trying new foods, tasting the foods that will be served at an upcoming gathering, serving themselves small portions if they will be required to finish their plate, and using utensils in a certain way. You might also practice role-playing the scenario they are about to face, whether that's saying *no thank you* to a meal or reacting to comments about their body. Regardless of your approach, help your child understand that they are learning these skills to help them navigate a tricky situation. If you suspect that your child thinks they've done something wrong, be very clear that this is not the case.

Some skills take a long time to master. Your child may or may not be able to master certain skills in the amount of time that you have before an upcoming event. If your child doesn't feel ready to use the new skills they've been working on, let them know that they shouldn't feel guilty. If your child is expected to be on their best behavior or use their new skills in a stressful situation, give them a day with fewer demands before and after the event. They also may be totally exhausted after using them, so expect more meltdowns.

PAUSE VISITS

Sometimes the other adults in your life won't budge and you might believe your child is being harmed in the process. Whether your objection is to an unsafe diet, lack of safety practices (like foods that are choking hazards), or, in the case of Lydia and Sofia, talking about your child's size or weight, it may be serious enough that you decide you need to pause on gathering with these people. If that's the case, use *I* language when delivering the news: "*Lydia and Sofia need to have space away from any talk about their bodies, so I'm going to come to the next gathering but leave them at home.*" Don't make it about them and everything they are doing wrong. Instead, talk about what your child needs and how taking a break will help them. Let the other person know that you're going to take a short break, and if the concerning behavior stops, you can start visiting again. This will help them understand that you want to keep the relationship open, but you are very serious about your concerns.

If pausing visits altogether is too extreme for your situation, you might be able to simply change the timing of your visits. If stress points are happening mostly during meals—such as someone commenting on what or how much your child is eating—visit outside of eating time.

PREPARE YOUR CHILD FOR THE SITUATION AND REFRAME IT FOR THEM

In some situations, there may be no way to enforce a boundary, and you can't remove the child from the situation. They may be exposed to perspectives on food that you would rather they not hear. In these cases, you may need to address it with the child ahead of time and discuss how they can best navigate the situation on their own. Your explanation of how to handle this will vary based on your child's age and comprehension, but might sound something like, "It's not okay to talk about other people's bodies without their permission. We know that bodies come in all shapes and sizes, and that is good, but some people think bigger sizes are bad. Sometimes Grandma and the aunties think this. It is sad and hurtful. It's not okay. If they say anything about your body, you can come tell me so we can talk about it."

If you know your child is going to be required to clean her plate, you might prep them by saying, "The rule at the Davidsons' house is that everyone must eat all the food on their plate before they can have dessert. This is not what our family does, but different families do different things. When you put food on your plate, put a small amount on at first so that you don't have a big pile of food on your plate if you're feeling full. You can always ask for a little bit more if you're still hungry."

Here are some scripts for explaining that some differences are okay or that people can be wrong about some things:

> "We do it this way, but that family does it that way. That's okay."
>
> "That isn't a good fit for our family, so here's how we can make it work better for us."
>
> "We love them and they are right about some things, but also we know that what they are saying about weight hurts people and isn't okay at all."

If you know your child will be exposed to hurtful language in a particular situation, explain to them beforehand that it is not okay for an adult to speak this way (assuming that this is age appropriate). You might also let your child know what you are doing to try to keep the harmful talk from happening. Also, be prepared to help your child process their experience afterward by asking what it was like, how they felt, and listening over the course of one or many conversations. If they are upset by the hurtful language, validate with them that it makes sense to be upset in this situation. Phrases that may be useful as part of conversations include:

"I hear you saying ____ happened."
"I heard Auntie say something to you about your body."
"What was that like?"
"You're right. It's not okay they did that."
"It makes sense that it feels bad when that happened. That was unfair."

HIGH-RISK STRATEGIES TO AVOID

If your child is facing a high-risk exposure, even if it's from someone you are close to, it is risky to ignore or downplay it. It can be extremely uncomfortable to confront family and friends about these issues, and it's often much easier to let it slide. However, hearing comments about the size or shape of their body, negative or positive, can have immediate and lifelong effects on children. Physically force-feeding and harsh punishments related to food can make a child's eating worse and can be traumatic for kids of any age. These practices can lead to a child having less respect for their body, as well as their hunger and fullness cues. Failing to observe tier 1 nutrition priorities can also be life-threatening. Just as these are high-risk activities for people to be using with a child, it is just as high risk for us to ignore them.

APPLYING THE SIX-STEP FRAMEWORK FOR SOFIA AND LYDIA

Step 1: Separate fact from fiction. Sofia and Lydia's mom struggled with her relatives' unwillingness to consider how their actions were affecting the girls. It was easy to decide that they were just being selfish and didn't really care about the kids. She was also tempted to think, *The girls will be fine*, since everyone in their family had grown up with similar talk surrounding weight. However, the girls' mom took the time to recognize both notions for what they were—stories she was telling herself—and decided to stick with the fact that what the girls were hearing wasn't helpful. They needed her advocacy, regardless of what anyone else in the family was thinking.

Step 2: Pick the priority. Sofia and Lydia's mom listed her priorities: her own comfort with the situation, the larger well-being of the family, her girls' relationship with their bodies, and more. In the end, she decided the top priority was protecting the girls' relationship with their bodies by reducing their exposure to weight stigma and body shaming.

Step 3: Brainstorm—with a twist. Their mom considered the following options: not attending family gatherings with the kids, talking to her family members about the issue, talking to the girls about the issue, and not changing anything (which she noted would be the same as choosing to let weight talk continue).

Step 4: Take a risk reduction approach. Sofia and Lydia's mom knew that by deciding to act, she would have a difficult conversation ahead that would potentially stress the relationship with her family. They tended to view the well-being of the extended family as top priority, so asking for a big change from the family for the sake of her kids was breaking with tradition and unlikely to be welcome. She knew her mom preferred to talk on the phone and that she would likely benefit from several weeks' notice before the family event. She also decided not to make any big threats (like, "We won't be able to do any family events if you can't get on board with this"), but to keep this first conversation positive and to be careful not to accuse her mother of anything.

Step 5: Think like a scientist and start an experiment. Sofia and Lydia's mom gave Grandma a call. This is how it went:

Mom: "Hi! The kids are so excited for next weekend and all the food! . . . I need to bring up one thing ahead of time. It's important for Sofia and Lydia that no one discusses their body size or shape in front of them. Sofia is saying negative things about her body, and Lydia may be thinking them."
Grandma: "You're just being sensitive. We talk about everyone's weight. We talked about your weight, and you turned out fine. Plus, Sofia is getting chubby, and it doesn't look good. She needs to hear that she should take it easy with her eating."
Mom: [*Ignores the "chubby" bait*] "I know we talk a lot about weight. For Lydia and Sofia, though, it's not safe. We can't let them hear this kind of talk if they are going to keep attending big gatherings. I'm happy to hear about your diet, though. Can we talk about it when the kids are all playing outside? Or can I call tomorrow?"
Grandma: [*insert critical comments about their parenting choices and lack of commitment to the extended family*]
Mom: [*ignores the critical comments*] "It's time for me to go now. We'll see you this weekend. Thanks, Mom."

Although the girls' mom did not get agreement and approval from Grandma, she did get her point across. Knowing that Grandma had not agreed to stop making comments about Sofia's body, Sofia's mom talked to Sofia about how Grandma and other family members often use words that are hurtful and wrong. They planned for Sofia to walk away if someone says something about Sofia's body.

The next weekend, after sending the girls out to play, Sofia and Lydia's mom called her mother to ask specifically about her weight-loss experiences, making it easier for them to not discuss diets in front of the kids. At the next family gathering following the phone call, when she notices Grandma is about to make a negative comment about Sofia's body, she boldly interrupts. Grandma gives her a painfully disapproving look but does not continue to comment on Sofia's size. Later that day, a relative makes a comment about Sofia's size, and Mom and Sofia walk away together.

Step 6: Celebrate your wins, then continue to tweak your experiment. After the event, the girl's mom assessed the experience. First, she patted herself on the back for all of the things she did to prepare for the event, and then made the difficult decision to have the girls play at a friend's house during the next family gathering. She called Grandma and other relatives ahead of time and, as gently and kindly as she could, explained that the girls wouldn't be able to attend because their bodies were repeatedly being discussed. They will try again in a few months. This is not a popular decision and causes a lot of hard feelings initially. The next time the girls are at a family event, however, no one in the family says anything about their bodies.

8

STARTING THE EATING JOURNEY

One of the earliest feeding decisions you will make regarding your child—perhaps only after the questions of breast milk, formula, or a combination—will be about starting to feed your child solid foods. A friend of mine who runs an animal rescue texted me about it a couple of years ago:

Just curious, what do you suggest for my daughter's first real food?

Oooooh, I can totally walk you through first foods. Want to do a video call?

Nah, I wean dogs and cats all the time. I mash up some food with liquid and start them there. I was planning to do the same thing with the baby. Which food should I mash up first?

I'd focus on high-iron foods... meat, beans, etc. Add a sprinkle of lemon or lime to most meals so she gets more iron.

Okay.

My friend's daughter is a preschooler now, and she's doing just fine. Although there are whole books and courses on how to start serving your child solid foods, believe it or not, figuring out how to start solid foods can be as simple as exchanging a few text messages.

However, a lot of us overthink this milestone. As parents, we have created some false obstacles for ourselves when it comes to getting babies to eat "real" food. Introducing solid foods is the start of a new adventure with your child, not a problem to solve. And yet we have come up with strict rules and "sides" that you can take in the baby feeding debate. But guess what? You don't have to pick a side. Instead, you can choose to stay above the fray and determine the best way of introducing solid foods to your baby by using the six-step process outlined in chapter 6.

Another name for gradually introducing solid foods alongside breast milk or formula is *complementary feeding*. People do this in a few ways. One method, baby-led weaning, involves introducing solid food to your child by letting them feed themselves finger foods instead of being spoon-fed. You've also likely come across plans for progressing from smooth purees to finger foods or "table foods" (foods *you* eat), which I like to call "puree to table" feeding. You've probably also come across hybrids of these plans. Sometimes these methods are presented with very strong claims attached to them, such as "Baby-led weaning prevents picky eating" or "Purees are more developmentally appropriate than finger foods." These can also can sound like, "Your baby will be picky if you don't use baby-led weaning," or "If you don't do baby-led weaning, you're not adequately preparing your baby for a lifetime of happy eating," or "You're ignoring your baby's developmental needs if you don't start with purees."

Often, as a result of these claims, I observe parents becoming emotionally invested in following one of these specific methods to a T or relying heavily on someone else's recommendation before knowing the needs of their individual child. Instead of trying to force-fit one of these methods, I encourage you to remain flexible in your mindset and to think about starting solid foods as an experiment.

As it turns out, all methods can be great methods for introducing solid foods, depending on the baby. So feel free to choose whatever method seems to work best, or pick and choose different parts of different methods to meet your child's needs. Current research does not support the idea that one is "better" than the others. Begin with the method that sounds interesting and fun to you, and be open to changing your strategy at any time. The first six months of feeding babies solid food is important, but it's not going to guarantee anything about your child's future. You don't have to be afraid of "ruining" your child because you didn't do baby-led weaning or puree feeding. Even if you really have your heart set on doing solids in one particular way, stay flexible—sometimes we're up against challenges and we need to do things that weren't our first choice, but we can still do a great job.

For some babies, the solid-foods phase can be a bit dicey, and for others, it can go just as planned. In either case, try to be flexible with the logistics so that you can enjoy the good parts. Yes, this is a time when eating concerns could show up and feeding in general gets "tricky" (because now you are actually feeding). But this is also the start of delightful moments when your baby beams with pride when they get a smashed blueberry into their mouth and everyone is connecting in a way that only eating together provides. Those are the times to focus on.

Daphne

Daphne is the youngest of three sisters, with two adoring older siblings who gave her parents plenty of experience moving babies from liquids to solid foods. Daphne's dad had been extremely picky as a child, and both parents wanted to avoid that at all costs with their first two, so they researched feeding methods and went all in on baby-led weaning. They took a course, following all the rules perfectly. They started their older daughters with safely sized and textured chunks of solid foods, and the girls were immediately into it. They progressed quickly, and there are two matching photos of the girls on the wall from when they were each around eighteen months, both wearing huge grins and spaghetti in their hair and sauce all over their faces. By four and six years old, respectively, the two older girls had begun eating like champs, with plenty of variety in their diets.

From infancy, Daphne had issues with feeding. Lactation consultants, pumping, combination feeding formula and breast milk, and alarms to make sure she ate enough were all part of her early feeding story. Her parents were looking forward to starting baby-led weaning and putting the early days behind them. The day she turned six months old, she was showing all the signs of being ready to eat, and the whole family gathered around the table as they offered her a safely prepared chicken drumstick. She refused to touch it and started crying. They tried again the next day, this time with an avocado slice coated in hemp seeds. They tried cooked oatmeal on a spoon, egg, safely prepared toast with nut butter, and more. Daphne became more and more upset at mealtimes, would barely touch anything, and would always end up crying. A few weeks in, her parents started to get concerned and they wondered what they were doing wrong this time around. Feeding Daphne was not going as expected.

WHAT'S GOING ON?

Most babies start out interested in eating. Between the ages of six and nine months, they are in an exploratory phase of life—a special window of time during which their brains are being trained to eat the flavors available to them. Babies who are ready to eat have control of their heads and necks, are interested in food and eating, sit alone (or with support), aren't reflexively pushing things out of their mouths with their tongues, and are bringing objects to their mouths. This usually happens around five or six months of age, and these babies usually accept most new foods readily, are willing to touch food and get messy, and put food in their mouths. They can start eating purees or safely prepared finger foods. Regardless of which foods they start with, they should progress in variety and texture as quickly as the baby can, eating at least some textured table foods by about eight to nine months old.

This isn't always how feeding goes, however. Things might not be working if your child has not progressed to textured table foods like mashed sweet potato or beans, soft cooked vegetables (squishable between forefinger and thumb), or meat run through a baby food mill by eight months old (if you are doing puree-to-table feeding), or if they continue to refuse to touch food or feed themselves after a few weeks of baby-led weaning. If your baby regularly gets upset at the sight of food, cries at the idea of eating, frequently gags or vomits when they try to eat, doesn't know what to do with food in their mouth, or eats only smooth foods or foods with a specific texture (such as only eating crunchy foods or dry foods that melt in the mouth like "puffs"), they might need a different strategy. Finally, if they refuse to touch foods or get their hands dirty, reject entire food groups, or are not gaining weight appropriately or are falling off their own growth curve, it is prudent to contact a healthcare provider promptly.

If any of these things happen, it does not mean you did anything wrong or used the wrong weaning method. These things happen to both puree-fed and finger food–fed babies. But rather than continuing down the path you're on, you might consider a different one. Sometimes parents continue on the path they're on despite red flags because of messages such as "Babies will eat when they're ready" (true, but if they aren't ready when expected, they may miss an important developmental window if it's not explored) or "They need teeth before they can progress beyond purees" (not true) or "Gagging is normal" (it can be, but excessive gagging and frequent vomiting are not and can trigger lasting eating issues) or "Your child will eat the right amount for them" (most can, but if they are not gaining, they aren't). When you keep an eye out for what is happening with your child, you can keep from getting distracted by "universal statements" and make changes as needed.

START WITH THE BASICS

The feeding practices in part 1 are helpful for starting to feed your baby solid foods on the right foot while keeping you flexible. They can be used whether you are using baby-led weaning, puree-to-table feeding, or a combination of the two.

As we've discussed, teaching your child to eat with embodied independence is about preserving their connection to their hunger and fullness cues, and giving them the tools they need to eat a variety of foods now and in the future. This can start from a very early age—from the time a child starts eating. One technique for beginning to teach your child about eating with embodied independence from a very young age is self-feeding, which involves letting your child feed themselves all or most of the time. The baby-led weaning method that Daphne's parents used relies solely on this, but self-feeding can be practiced with puree-to-table feeding as well. Allowing your baby to self-feed makes it relatively easy to know when they are full, because they will stop eating (or start throwing) the food, and getting food all over themselves helps their body learn to tolerate new textures and sensations, which paves the way for eating more textures. It also builds hand-eye coordination and fine motor development.

You can still practice elements of self-feeding, even if you are holding the spoon while feeding your child purees, by becoming more observant and making sure they are opening their mouth on their own and leaning their head forward, indicating they want more food. That old airplane game, where you pretend the spoon with food is an airplane to get a baby to open their mouth and eat, tends to work against their sense of embodiment, but holding a spoon out so that they can choose to put their head forward to take a bite *builds* their sense of embodiment.

When babies are first born, it's recommended that you feed them on demand whenever they show hunger and fullness cues. When you start solid foods, however, you can move right into an eating routine that will slowly become their meal and snack routine. Most babies don't need snacks. By age one, they will usually be eating three meals a day and may also still be having breast milk or formula. As a result, you can start to be mindful about whether you're using food to fix emotions or boredom (and potentially adjust that tendency) when they are quite young. This is also the time to be firm about setting the menu as the parent. If your baby doesn't eat what's offered, don't bring a different food; just stick with your original offering. This sets the stage for the toddler phase to help them know what to expect and for you to practice holding your boundaries.

Embodiment also entails exposing babies to a variety of textures and flavors to help them develop a tolerance for flavors and texture variety as mentioned above. This will help them to eat more variety and to meet their nutrient needs in the future. Personally, I found it easy to start with the textured purees that come out of a simple baby food mill (a little hand crank at the table) to get the texture train going. Other parents like to start with baby-led-weaning-style finger foods or something smoothly pureed. However you choose to start, the goal is getting your child to table foods (foods eaten by the rest of the family during meals) as quickly as is safely possible. Stay curious and keep testing their ability to branch out to more complex textures.

For many years, it was commonly recommended to introduce one food to babies at a time to observe for allergic reactions. New research, however, has changed consensus recommendations, which include feeding an infant a diverse diet and not delaying the introduction of potentially allergenic foods. Unless your healthcare provider has recommended otherwise for medical reasons, you can introduce multiple foods at once to expand the diversity of your baby's diet. And don't forget about bitter and savory flavors. One trend right now is to serve your baby one hundred different foods by the age of one. If that sounds fun to you, go for it! It can be a great way to make sure you introduce a variety of flavors. If that sounds like another demand on your mental energy (it did to me when I was feeding my babies), just feed them whatever you're eating to get the variety in. You don't need to expose them to any foods you don't usually eat just to get to one hundred foods. I've never seen a research study about one hundred foods—there's nothing magical about that number from a health standpoint.

Babies can join the table, too! Pull their seat up to the table and let them be part of the fun. This has the added benefit of exposing a child to more foods and giving them the chance to be in on the excitement and connection of dinnertime. They'll also see an adult modeling eating different foods. When my kids were babies, my favorite setup was to make dinner, sit down to the meal, and give the baby some of our food. If the meal wasn't baby-friendly, I'd pop it into that little hand grinder and let them feed themselves a textured puree of dinner. Eating together made this easy and contributed to the variety of flavors that babies benefit from. It's also a great time to start building the habit of family meals if you haven't already. If your baby goes to bed before your dinnertime, see if you can sit down and eat with them at a different time.

When your child is a baby, this is a perfect time for parents to start practicing the mindset that they want to cultivate in their child. This could include thinking about which messages you want to convey to your child, considering how you want to use the words *healthy* or *unhealthy*, and practicing talking about foods factually. You can point out the names of different foods to the baby as you model eating them. Anything you hope to say (or not say) to your kids about food—start now! It's never too early, and the more you practice, the more natural it will become.

Because their stomachs are tiny and because they are going through a unique developmental period, babies have nutrient needs that are different from those of older children. The most important nutrients for babies to have are iron, zinc, calcium, vitamin D, vitamin C (to help with iron absorption), choline, protein, and fat. Fish, beans and legumes, tofu, dark green veggies, eggs, plain yogurt, fortified cereals, red meat, poultry, and liver are all food items that contain many of these nutrients in one food, so they make great foods to focus on at the beginning. You might start off with iron-fortified oatmeal offered on a spoon, bean soup puree offered on a spoon with some lime sprinkled on it, or tofu strips and a large, soft strawberry (bigger than the baby's mouth) or well-mashed strawberries on a spoon. Other options for getting these important nutrients in include: a piece of lightly toasted bread about two finger-lengths in width with a thin spread of peanut butter or mashed egg on it; or cooked ground beef, poultry, or fish, prepared for self-feeding (such as a chicken drumstick baked with skin, tendons, and all nonmeat parts removed). A vitamin D supplement is usually recommended for babies receiving human milk.

Introducing the top allergens, such as dairy, soy, egg, peanuts, tree nuts, and wheat, early in the weaning process is also a best practice. Not only are these foods nutritious, but eating them often as a baby has been associated with lower risk of developing allergies. If you have concerns about allergies or introducing common allergens, speak with your child's healthcare provider.

It's important to note that there are some foods that are not safe for babies. Watch out for choking hazards, and modify anything hard, round, slippery, or chewy. These include whole grapes, grape tomatoes, berries, cherries, melon balls, pieces of kernel corn, and canned fruit; pieces of hard, raw fruits and veggies; uncooked dry fruit (like raisins); whole, chopped, thick spread nuts / nut butters; chunks of meat or cheese / string cheese; fish with bones; hot dogs, meat sticks, and sausages; cookies and granola bars; chips, pretzels, and crackers; bread with seeds or nuts; hard candy, jelly beans, gummies, marshmallows; gum; and popcorn. Honey is not safe until age one because it can cause botulism. Raw or undercooked fish, meat, dairy, or eggs and high-sodium seasonings should also be avoided.

When it comes to structured permission, babyhood is the "delay" phase. They don't know what they are missing, even if they are curious about it. This is the time to eat your chocolate in peace while they are taking a nap (unless it's just me who thinks chocolate tastes so much better when the kids are asleep).

See how long you can delay introducing added sugars or other hyperpalatable foods. The goal for added sugars is delaying for two years and delaying other hyperpalatable foods for "as long as you can" (which may not be two years), as this can potentially lower later-life disease risk. Also see how long you can delay juice and other sweet beverages. If delaying hyperpalatable foods affects *your* personal relationship with food or your body, or it doesn't work with your lifestyle or finances, then you can modify. The overarching goal is to get babies the most exposure possible to plain, non-hyperpalatable foods so that their palates are trained on these and so that they can get the nutrition that they need during this critical period.

Also, I know it can be a real slog to always be focusing on choking hazards and chopping up some foods and delaying others, but these phases do end! It's one reason I give recommendations for how long to do something. For example, sometimes it's easier to follow "No juice until two" instead of "Delay juice as long as possible," because you know it will end at a specific time. I had this mindset when it came to preventing choking hazards, and I know I'm not the only one. "Just two more years and I'll be out of grape-cutting jail," one mom with a two-year-old told me.

PROBLEM-SOLVING STRATEGIES TO TRY

If you find your baby is not progressing as expected when it comes to starting to eat solid foods, something may be up. It may be time to consider one of the strategies below.

TRY A DIFFERENT METHOD

Curiosity is essential for weaning. When I started feeding my first son at six months old, I mixed breast milk with mashed banana and tried to feed it to him on a spoon. I thought I was going to feed him with the spoon initially, then he would smear pureed banana all over his face, and then we would slowly work toward him feeding himself. But he grabbed the spoon out of my hand and managed to feed himself his first bite of food. He was insistent about feeding himself from day one. I had to follow his lead and thicken purees and prepare finger foods because he would rather poke himself in the eye with a spoon full of mashed yams than have us feed him. Although I didn't know about different weaning methods, I was able to meet him where he was by using curiosity.

I find parents have an easier time transitioning from puree-to-table feeding to a self-feeding approach, if purees weren't going well, rather than from baby-led weaning to purees. There seems to be a lot more guilt and emotional angst over stopping baby-led weaning. Parents, like Daphne's, say they are afraid their baby will become an extreme picky eater, they don't like having to give up "the best" method of feeding, or they feel like a failure if they couldn't do it "right." I can understand how parents might feel that way given the exaggerated promises and fear-based messaging that we see on social media and in some books surrounding baby-led weaning.

If you do find your child really struggling with baby-led weaning, it's possible they already have a tendency to eating problems, and "failing" at baby-led weaning has nothing to do with you and everything to do with the internal hurdles your child has that you are just learning about. This is the time to embrace courage, make changes, and start incorporating different methods of weaning to help your baby progress with eating in a way that they can handle so that they can continue to progress.

CHECK IN WITH A HEALTHCARE PROVIDER

If you suspect something isn't quite right with your child's eating, check in with their healthcare provider. This is especially true if they aren't eating some solid foods by the time they are eight months old.

HIGH-RISK STRATEGIES TO AVOID

IGNORING THE PROBLEM

If your baby isn't progressing as expected with solid foods, it's not the time to ignore the issue. It's not time to panic either. It's time to engage. Ignoring eating problems early can make eating problems bigger sooner. The most common situation I hear is parents who say, "I was told that with baby-led weaning, the baby would start eating when they were ready and I didn't need to worry about it, so I didn't think about how much time was passing." This "start when they're ready" advice has a grain of truth, but it's better to get involved early than late when it comes to feeding challenges.

FORCE-FEEDING

Force-feeding is a negative experience that not only works against your child's embodiment but can create long-term negative associations with mealtime, which can make future feeding much harder.

APPLYING THE SIX-STEP FRAMEWORK FOR DAPHNE

Now let's return to Daphne's story and look at how her parents might use the six-step framework introduced at the start of part 2 to problem-solve for her feeding dilemma.

Step 1: Separate fact from fiction. Daphne's parents needed to get to the bottom of what was really going on, beyond blaming themselves for what they may or may not have been doing "wrong." Daphne's two older sisters had been great eaters. Were they not giving Daphne the time and attention she needed, because now they were juggling the responsibilities of three children? Daphne's parents had doubts about their parenting, but they quickly reality-checked that story and put it to the side. They noted that Daphne seemed to have had eating troubles from the start, separate from the time they put in or whatever approach they tried.

Step 2: Pick the priority. Daphne's parents considered their time, the family dynamics with their other daughters, Daphne's nutrition, and Daphne's developmental eating skills. Given her age and developmental window, they decided the first priority was to make sure Daphne could progress in her eating skills.

Step 3: Brainstorm—with a twist. Daphne's parents made a list of actions they could take, listed their pros and cons, and eventually landed on contacting Daphne's healthcare provider for assessment and advice. They also decided that they would immediately stop baby-led weaning and try puree feeding instead, to see if she had a better response to that method. They also had the idea to include Daphne's older sisters more in feeding. Daphne adored them as much as they adored her, and the parents thought Daphne might be more willing to copy or eat when they were involved.

Step 4: Take a risk reduction approach. Daphne's parents recognized that puree feeding might not give Daphne the same experiences of embodiment if they were feeding her with a spoon, so after making a list of risk reduction items, they decided to give her an option of feeding herself with a spoon and putting her head forward and opening her mouth to have her parents or siblings feed her. They made sure to show their older daughters what that looked like, since they would be helping feed their baby sister. They also decided they would do whatever possible to make mealtime fun.

Step 5: Think like a scientist and start an experiment. While they waited for the appointment with Daphne's healthcare provider, her parents began to offer smooth purees using their risk reduction approach of allowing Daphne to feed herself. They offered iron-fortified baby oatmeal on a spoon, and they found that when Daphne's sisters fed her, she was willing to eat the oatmeal and loved her sisters cheering for her! She still was unwilling to feed herself, however. Nevertheless, they were encouraged by the positive experience and began offering Daphne a variety of pureed vegetables and meats with her sisters as her cheering squad, which proved successful. Later they met with Daphne's healthcare provider, who suggested an assessment by a pediatric speech language pathologist to determine whether Daphne might need support with oral-motor or sensory system development.

Step 6: Celebrate your wins, then continue to tweak your experiment. Daphne's parents congratulated all the kids at mealtime—for having fun, feeding each other, and trying new foods. They also congratulated each other for being willing to change course when their child needed it, even though they were in unknown territory. They knew they would get more information from Daphne's upcoming assessment and they might need to change things, so they adopted a flexible mindset for the feeding journey ahead.

9

MEALTIME MADNESS, FROM TABLE MANNERS TO FOOD BATTLES

Splat. A piece of watermelon hit our friend in the face, and our son, who was one at the time, delighted in the accuracy of his aim. My husband and I apologized profusely, and our friend had a good sense of humor about it, but we were less than thrilled with his newfound dinnertime "skill."

Eating together as a family is one of the core pillars of our plan, but when it comes to managing kid behavior, family meals can sometimes feel like a battleground. You've finally gotten your child to eat solid foods, but now you are dealing with children who bring their own set of challenges. From spilled milk and clothes covered in ketchup, to food throwing and Houdini-esque attempts to escape the high chair, mealtime can raise blood pressure even if you know it's an activity that will benefit the family.

Malik, Maya, and Kai

The Jackson parents have three kids: three-year-old twins Malik and Maya, and baby Kai, who just turned one. The Jacksons are emerging from the "survival" phase of raising an infant and two young toddlers, a time when mealtimes were complete chaos, and table manners weren't even a consideration. Kai has just learned to throw food, and no one has time to clean his spaghetti off the wall. Malik is a wonderfully independent kid who likes to stand on his chair and declare, "I don't like this, I won't eat it," which triggers a battle of his parents negotiating with him and pressuring him to eat. Maya is an active kid who does not like to stop running around to sit down to a meal. Once her parents finally get her to the table, she's up and in another room before they can even start eating. The parents are over it and want to have meals that feel more positive. At least one of them has lost their cool several times in the past week because family meals are so stressful. They want to turn the situation around, but with three kids, all with different needs, they are unsure of the best approach.

WHAT'S GOING ON?

We may not realize it, but mealtime asks a lot of kids. For a child, it takes energy and focus to sit and eat—plus, if that child is picky, tired, or learning a new skill, they may not be bringing their best self to the table. This is true whether the child is one year old or eleven (and frankly, when I've had a long day, sometimes I don't bring my best self to dinner either).

If you're new to the dinnertime chaos game, welcome. A few lucky parents win the "perfectly behaved child at mealtime" lottery, but for most of us, meals with our kids are occasionally, if not always, a circus. Some kids grow out of mealtime madness quickly, while others keep coming up with new ways to keep the mayhem going.

START WITH THE BASICS

If you struggle with hectic family meals, as a start, I suggest that you focus on the second and third pillars in the first part of this book: eating with embodied independence and eating together. These are foundational practices, and when we help kids learn to listen to their bodies and connect with the people around them, sometimes better behavior at mealtimes reveals itself. However, if after concentrating on these two principles your child still exhibits problem behaviors at mealtime, you'll need more targeted strategies.

PROBLEM-SOLVING STRATEGIES TO TRY

When one of our sons was eighteen months old, he threw a mug from the table, and it shattered on the floor. Our bad for giving him something breakable, knowing he loved to throw his cups. All his other mealtime behaviors were great: He sat in his seat, tried new foods, engaged in family meals, used age-appropriate utensils, drank out of an open cup, and he didn't throw food. But when it came to throwing cups, we tried all the common-sense strategies we could think of (like not giving it back after it was thrown), then we talked to everyone we knew and tried their strategies (like throwing a ball for five minutes before the meal). No dice. He just *loved* throwing his cup. After months of trying to fix this problem, we decided it wasn't hurting anyone, there were other more important things for us to put our parenting energy into, and we just waited for him to grow out of it, which he did (and now his sports teams appreciate how well he can throw).

I do remember feeling very frustrated about the cup throwing while it was happening. Now that I know the end of the story, though—that he grew out of it and his baseball teams loved him—I think it's funny. It always makes me smile, and I love that it happened. All of that to say, the strategies in this chapter may work for you, but if they don't, take heart—you may just be rewarded with a memory that makes you smile for the rest of your life.

This chapter has lots of common-sense strategies that I've gleaned from personal experience, friends' experiences, and input from specialists. I think of this section as a conversation we'd have at the playground while pushing our kids on the swings and trading ideas for dealing with our little mealtime annoyances. "Have you tried . . . ?" "This worked for us. . . ." You know kids. They have minds of their own, and what works for one child doesn't necessarily work for another. These suggestions are a great place to start as you look to solve problems with less risky and more creative strategies.

REJECT FOOD BATTLES

The fastest way out of a food battle is to just . . . not engage. You don't actually have to battle your child at mealtime.

When Malik says, "I'm not going to eat that."

His parents could say, "You don't have to; just sit with us."

Refusing to engage takes the wind out of a child's sails because there's nothing to push back on. You opted out of the battle. Based on my observations, a kid who announces that they don't like a meal, or won't eat it, will often eat that meal if the parent says, "Okay." Try sitting there for five minutes, without pressuring them and pretending that you don't care. Chances are, your kid will get in touch with their feeling of hunger and decide to eat anyway.

Saying okay when a kid refuses to eat requires tolerating a kid who isn't eating. If you're using one-bite rules and it's leading to food battles, that may be your sign that one-bite rules aren't a great fit for your family.

DON'T TAKE COMPLAINTS PERSONALLY

"You never make anything that I like. You know I don't like this meal. You don't love me."

I almost laughed out loud when my son said this to me. Of course I make things he likes. He had eaten this exact beef stew two weeks prior with no complaints. And of course, he knows I love him. He'd had a rough day at school, though, he was tired, and it's true that this particular dinner was not his favorite. That's really all he was saying.

I do not take comments about dinner personally (99 percent of the time). We work with our kids on not speaking negatively about food or complaining about it, especially to the person who cooked it. But when complaints or critiques inevitably come up, even if I spent two hours making the meal, I try to let it roll off my back (this is why I don't spend two hours making meals). They're kids. They'd be less likely to complain if they had experienced food insecurity, so this is actually a good thing in some ways. They don't know how good they have it—someone buying and making all their food and snacks for them every day. They aren't trying to offend me, they are still learning to think before they speak. Sometimes I think very negative thoughts about food before I eat it, too; I've just learned not to say them.

If we take complaints and picky eating personally, it adds a lot of unnecessary angst to our lives and makes feeding kids harder. It also may make us more likely to pressure a child to eat or finish their plate, thus leading to more upset during mealtime. This is one area where choosing *how* we react can make a big difference in whether a mealtime is pleasant or not.

MAKE IT EASIER FOR KIDS TO COME TO THE TABLE

Getting kids to come to dinner (or any meal) can be a battle for all sorts of reasons. Some kids do not want to stop doing what they are doing. Other kids just don't like the eating experience. Your kid may have their own reason, one that may or may not make sense to you.

To make things easier for kids who just don't love dinner, start by establishing a premeal routine. Knowing that a certain set of actions will always happen before the meal, and always in the same order, can help get kids in the mindset for meals. Your premeal routine could be as simple as washing hands, setting the table together, and sitting down.

Another way to make mealtime easier for kids, like Maya, who don't want to stay at the table is to make it fun. Try playing I spy, twenty questions, or a card game like Uno or Go Fish. Try doing family taste tests, which I describe in chapter 10. Take turns reading from a joke book. Do something that makes trying new foods together more fun, like introducing a new food or dish at dinner every day and then deciding on your family's favorite at the end of the week. You might also try serving dessert with dinner, rather than after dinner. This is a way to avoid bribing kids with sweets to eat dinner, and it can lower the hype surrounding certain foods (though I should point out that it works for some kids and not others—some might still obsess over the dessert or refuse to eat dinner after eating it). As long as you're not using dessert as a reward for coming to the table, and instead just making it part of their meal, this practice can be a positive motivator. Finally, make sure your kids are hungry at mealtime. If they aren't, they will be much less likely to want to quit whatever they are doing to come eat.

As discussed in part 1, if mealtimes are consistently a negative experience, it might be best to consider a pause on family meals for the time being. Sometimes family meals just aren't the best option. If that's the case for you, it may be better for everyone to eat separately when they are hungry.

TEACH MANNERS WITHOUT THE LECTURE

When I was about twelve, I remember my parents getting a book about manners. At family dinners, someone would read something out of the book, and then we would practice using that particular manner—even manners for formal occasions that we had never been a part of (like which fork to use if there were two). It was fun! Although I don't know what caused my parents to start the "manners initiative," I can only imagine them thinking at some point, *Things have gotten out of hand. We need some manners around here!* My younger siblings and I got lots of practice, and eventually, the manners book disappeared.

Recently, we decided to do a little manners boot camp at my house. We had the kids list out all the manners that should happen during mealtime, and then we made a game out of it. Everyone's manners (including my own) improved within a few nights.

Is it developmentally appropriate to teach table manners to toddlers? Sure! As long as you recognize that table manners will be a work in progress for years. Your toddler can start to learn to help set the table, wash their hands before meals, stay seated, say *please* and *thank you*, and not throw food. As kids get older, they can learn how to pass food, how to have conversations at the table, and how to listen to other people. They can learn not to talk with their mouths full and not to say anything bad about foods. But keep in mind that it may take time!

It may not work to teach manners in the heat of the moment at the dinner table. Instead, try practicing the manners you want your child to display when you're away from the table, with dolls or stuffies. "Lucy the duck says, 'Mommy, may I please have water?'" You can also practice with your child. "Let's pretend you have the corn and I really want more corn. I can say, 'Would you please pass the corn?'"

Don't take on too much at a time. Rather than expecting your child to learn all the manners at once, focus on one specific manner during a meal. "We're going to practice saying, 'Thank you,' during lunch today." You can make it light and fun, using silly voices to say *thank you* or playfully "catching" your child if they forget. Make sure to "forget" your manners occasionally so that they can catch you, too. Keeping things playful will make the experience more positive, even when you're working on a skill.

You can also use *labeled praise* to encourage polite behavior at the table. Labeled praise is telling your child what they did that you liked. It sounds like:

"You waited for everyone to be served before you started eating!"

"I noticed you said *thank you* to Auntie when she poured your water last night."

"You asked me to pass the butter instead of grabbing it. I bet you're proud of remembering that."

COMBAT TODDLER FOOD THROWING

This one starts with setting a boundary. When Kai throws a food, his parents can immediately hold his hand, tell him, "No," or "Food stays here," and end the meal for him. If you do this with your food thrower at home, they may be hungry soon if they weren't able to finish their meal, and if they are you can offer a snack, even if it's out of your routine. Then ask yourself why your child may be throwing food. Do they think it's a game and love the attention? Are they full and bored? Are they worried about a new food? Maybe they're distracted or just simply love throwing. The strategy you use to quash the food throwing will likely depend on the why. Below are some possible reasons why your toddler may be throwing food, along with recommended responses:

Your child thinks it's a game and loves the attention.

Don't react to the food throwing. Take the food away, clean up if needed, and do it all calmly and without the emotion. Then tell your child that it's time to leave the table—if food is thrown, the meal is over.

Your child is full and bored.

Assuming that your young toddler is throwing food because they have had enough to eat and are bored, teach them to say or use sign language to say, "All done!" Then as soon as they are done, let them get down from their chair. You might also shorten mealtime and let them get down sooner. It's possible your toddler may find it difficult to sit for twenty minutes if they are active. If you don't want to shorten mealtime, you can remove all food from their reach after they look like they are full.

As usual, make sure they are coming to the meal hungry. If your child is snacking all day, they may not be hungry at mealtime, in which case, they'll get bored of the food fast. Combat boredom by adding some fun to the meal by "playing" with your food to engage them so that they are less likely to throw it.

Your child is worried about the food.

If fear or nerves are the issue, give them a "place" to put the food they don't want. It could be a bowl or the table, or they can hand it back to you. Give them only tiny portions of new foods.

Your child loves throwing or just learned to throw.

Go outside and play catch with them with a ball before the meal to "get it out of their system." Then give them only one piece of food at a time so that there isn't "extra" for them to throw.

Your child isn't fully supported in their chair.

Put a pillow or blanket behind them so that they can sit up straight. If they don't have a footrest on their chair, put a band around the front two legs of their chair so that they have something to put their feet on, which helps them stabilize.

Some children who aren't fully supported in their chairs will move around to try to stabilize themselves. In this case, use the 90-90-90 sitting arrangement. Make sure they can put their feet on the floor, a box, or a footrest so that their knees are at a 90-degree angle. Make sure they have enough support that they can sit up straight with their back forming a 90-degree angle with the seat of the chair. And make sure they are sitting high enough that their elbows can be more or less at a 90-degree angle.

Even if your child loves mealtime, kids' attention spans vary. But you can help your child learn to sit for meals. Here is one method that has worked for my kids and many others.

1. Get a timer and set it for one minute per your child's years of age (I know this sounds like a tiny amount of time).

2. Make sure your child sits at the table until the timer goes off, even if you need to hug them on your lap to keep them there. Let them get down as soon as the timer goes off.
3. Increase the time they are required to sit at the table by a minute or two every day or every other day.
4. Increase the time until you reach their maximum attention span, the point at which they just cannot stay seated any longer. The length will vary by child.
5. Optional: Use a visual timer, such as a sand hourglass timer, a digital timer that your child can watch as the numbers count down, or a timer with hands where a colored section of the clock gets smaller as time progresses. This way, your child can reference it throughout meals in the future without constantly asking you, "How much time is left?" I like the sand timer because it's silent, and if they are having a good night and fun at the table, they sit longer.

UNDERSTAND APPROPRIATE UTENSIL USE

It is okay for kids to use their hands to eat. People eat with their hands all over the world. In some places, it's some of the time; in other places, it's almost all the time. Plus, when kids are touching foods, they are getting a sensory experience, which can help them learn to eat a wider variety of foods. The thing to be aware of is making sure they *can* use utensils. As long as your child is developing their ability to drink from cups and use a variety of utensils as a toddler, even if they aren't always successful or they choose not to, they are on the right track. If you find your child is never using their utensils and it is disrupting meals, then you may be able to work on it from a "manners" standpoint. If you think something else is going on with their development, you can check in with their healthcare provider.

HIGH-RISK STRATEGIES TO AVOID

EXPECTING PERFECTION AND MAKING MEALTIMES ENTIRELY ABOUT BEHAVIOR

The most significant risk to addressing mealtime behavior is making mealtimes a negative experience that everyone dreads. Since children are learning and some of them seem to constantly be finding new ways to bring madness to meals, you may always have something to "work on." If that's your focus and you're using punishments and constant corrections, it may create negative associations with mealtime. This doesn't mean you shouldn't address unacceptable behavior or hold boundaries, but it does mean giving everyone at the table a little bit of flexibility to be human.

APPLYING THE SIX-STEP FRAMEWORK FOR MALIK, MAYA, AND KAI

Step 1: Separate fact from fiction. The Jacksons' confidence in their parenting skills was at an all-time low. The mealtime chaos was overwhelming, and they thought if they were only better parents, their kids would be doing better. They pictured their children as teenagers, living a wildly chaotic life with no boundaries, and then as parents who wouldn't be able to handle their kids either. There were so many problems to fix—at some level, they were afraid to even try to improve things. They gave themselves a pep talk, though. Things were hard and had gotten out of hand, but they were engaged parents and they could start tackling the issues one by one.

Step 2: Pick the priority. The Jackson parents listed their priorities, which included ending the food throwing; making family meals less chaotic; supporting their kids' nutrition; helping their kids learn to listen to hunger and fullness cues; and one day being able to have guests over to the house for meals (which currently seemed impossible). They decided that a focus on "lowering the chaos" would be a good priority for them.

Step 3: Brainstorm—with a twist. One evening, the parents sat together and made a list of potential things they could try to lessen mealtime chaos. Possibilities included having the kids watch TV for meals, setting and holding new boundaries, and making some physical changes to the eating area and the way the kids were seated. They considered how each potential change might impact their own energy levels, whether the changes were even realistic, and how all three kids might react to each change. This wasn't a short conversation, but it felt good to talk through the different scenarios, and they had a short list of strategies to try.

Step 4: Take a risk reduction approach. The parents' biggest concern was that the new boundaries would make mealtimes even more negative and stressful than they already were. They were running on empty, and maybe they would give up on family meals altogether if they got any worse. They didn't have many concerns about the strategies themselves; it was the *how* that they thought was risky. To help with that, they decided to take on the smallest and easiest strategy first—improving the ergonomics of the kids' seating to give them more stability at the table—and to start it on a slow weekend, when they didn't have anything planned and there was less stress. Hopefully, that would give them the bandwidth they needed to do something extra at mealtimes without melting down themselves.

Step 5: Think like a scientist and start an experiment. To improve the kids' stability at the table, they started by getting diaper boxes and putting them under Malik's and Maya's feet. They also wrapped a band around the legs of Kai's high chair, so that all the kids had a place to put their feet and feel stable. They watched to see how long the kids sat and whether they left the table or not: Maya stopped getting down from the table, and often—and surprisingly—Kai's food throwing seemed to decrease a bit.

Step 6: Celebrate your wins, then continue to tweak your experiment. The Jacksons were proud of themselves for this win. It took some intentional time and effort to make it happen, but they had succeeded in making mealtimes less chaotic. This small win gave the parents a boost in their confidence, and they felt motivated to take on the next task. Despite the win, the food throwing was still unacceptable, and Malik was still standing up and demanding alternatives to most meals.

They decided to double down, hold boundaries, and stop responding to any invitations to mealtime drama. If Malik stands up and announces he's not going to eat spinach, they say, "Okay. You can have some rice." They are also very firm that they will not get up to offer or make anything else. At the same time, if Kai throws food, they immediately take him out of his chair and end his meal.

Initially, things felt chaotic again. Kai was hungry an hour after meals. Plus, Malik has refused to eat altogether after not getting what he wants, so now the parents are making a bedtime snack (when it's not part of their normal routine) and there is still mealtime drama. They had agreed to give it a few weeks, though, and within a few days, Kai stopped throwing food. Once he stopped throwing food, they stopped offering bedtime snack. It only took Malik a few more days to realize his parents weren't going to budge on making him a special meal, so he started going along with whatever was for dinner.

Mealtimes were still far from perfect with three kids aged three and under at the table. But the Jacksons were starting to have more enjoyable mealtime moments than drama moments—and that felt like a huge win.

10

TYPICAL PICKY EATING

My baby ate everything, then when she turned one, everything changed! Now she eats hardly anything and won't eat some of the foods she used to love," a mom messaged me one day.

There is no official definition of *picky eating*, but loosely defined, typical picky eating happens when a child won't just eat whatever you put in front of them. It's incredibly common, and it's likely you've encountered it in some form. Researchers use all sorts of definitions when studying this topic, but mine is "Whatever a parent thinks is picky"—because if your child isn't eating what you made and you feel frustrated, you need a name for it. If, on the other hand, your child has such a selective diet that it's disrupting the family's life, that would be considered extreme picky eating, which is discussed in chapter 11.

Gemma

Gemma just turned two and has transformed into a picky eater. She won't try new foods, and she's throwing foods she used to like at the wall. When she refuses to eat what she's given for a meal, she walks into the kitchen and points to the crackers that she does like, and if she doesn't get them, she lies on the floor and has a tantrum. Her parents are frustrated because they fed her a variety of foods as a baby and she was an adventurous eater. One of her parents thinks they need to push her to eat the foods she's refusing. The other parent thinks they should let her decide what she's going to eat and then give her a little snack later to make sure she's gotten enough to eat. They wonder if she's going to become pickier over time and worry that she's not getting the nutrition she needs.

WHAT'S GOING ON?

It's common for toddlers to start being choosy, nervous about new foods, and varying the amount of food they eat from one day to the next. Even babies who were introduced to a hundred foods before they turned one can become picky. Most typically, picky kids start being picky sometime after they turn one. With that said, despite their pickiness, these kids are still willing to eat foods from all the food groups, they can learn to eat new foods, and they tend to outgrow their pickiness within a few years. Keep in mind that picky eating isn't something that kids do to make their parents mad. When your child learns to talk and says they don't like dinner, they are just being a kid. Remember—what your child eats does not define your success as a parent!

Often what parents think of as "picky eating" is just the transition from baby energy needs to toddler energy needs. Your baby may have eaten like a professional athlete, but then suddenly, they enter toddlerhood and start eating like a bird. Babies often triple their birthweight in the first year of life. They are growing a lot! Toddlers only grow several inches. Still, this shift in what children eat—some days only a few bites—can be alarming and parents might assume it's due to pickiness rather than age-appropriate growth. The reality is that some kids just aren't that hungry (except when they are). Other kids will continue to eat heartily into toddlerhood, and that's fine, too. If your child is following their expected growth trajectories, then it's likely they're getting what they need. The problem with panicking about how much your child is eating is that you might swoop in with hyperpalatable foods or high-pressure tactics to try to get them to eat more. And these strategies can easily lead to more picky eating and long-term habits that are trickier to manage.

Early childhood is also when some of the causes of picky eating, such as sensory processing challenges, lack of interoception, or neurodivergence, start to present themselves. So, while picky eating is a common phase some kids go through, and most kids easily outgrow food neophobia (fear of new foods), for others, it's the beginning of a more difficult feeding journey. If you have concerns that your child's picky eating may be more serious or if you are wondering if they have risk factors for more serious eating problems, the Pediatric Screener for ARFID and Extreme Picky Eating (PSA-Eat) is a screening tool to provide healthcare providers and parents with useful information about their child's eating.

As kids get older, they may become pickier as they are exposed to more and more hyperpalatable foods that make "normal" foods seem boring or tasteless, or they may have negative experiences with foods that make them not want to eat it anymore.

START WITH THE BASICS

The feeding practices in part 1—eating with embodied independence, eating together, and eating without judgment, in particular—are helpful for keeping typical picky eating in check.

I mentioned this in chapter 2, but it bears repeating here: I've noticed that often, as is the case for Gemma, when a child has two caregivers, one caregiver is good at helping their child be "embodied" and another caregiver is good at teaching "independence." So, one parent forces a child to eat certain amounts of foods and never backs down from what they had planned on making for lunch, and the other parent lets the child decide how much they will eat, but if their child says they don't want something for dinner, the parent will get them something else. They both think the other person is doing it wrong. This can also be true in co-parenting and caregiver relationships. In reality, both people may be taking their strength a little too far and the child would benefit from more balance. You can use curiosity to find a strategy that both adults are comfortable with to start an experiment.

Also remember that it's not your job to make your child happy all the time. We make the mistake of thinking that *all* our mealtimes need to be happy and that if kids have any unhappiness around food, it will damage their relationship with food. This just isn't true. We do want positive mealtimes, and we want this most of the time. That doesn't mean we need to serve whatever kids want. It's okay for kids to be upset or uncomfortable with what we serve for dinner. Being firm about only serving one meal (while making sure there is at least one food they usually eat on the table), goes a long way in reducing picky eating. I know it's not always comfortable to have your child expressing how angry they are that you didn't make them the dinner they wanted. I've experienced this plenty. But I remind myself that I'm the parent, it's my job to set the menu, and my kids are allowed to be upset about it.

PROBLEM-SOLVING STRATEGIES TO TRY

Most of the strategies below for addressing your child's typical picky eating have few downsides. The main risk with them is that as parents, we become inflexible or overbearing about our approach, and we end up making mealtime a consistently negative experience. The exception to this is the "rewarding" strategy described below. It is a bit different in that it comes with some risks on its own. If you decide to use it, think about it from a risk reduction perspective to reduce potential harm.

TRY IT AGAIN

It can take kids many exposures to a food before they are willing to eat it. The best way forward with a child who has neophobia is to serve the foods until they are not new anymore. If you serve broccoli a couple of times a week for a year, it's definitely not new to them anymore. You don't have to put more on their plate than you know they could possibly eat, but do offer a micro-portion so that they can get used to the food—even if they don't eat it. When I say *micro-portion*, I mean: one pea, a piece of cabbage the size of your pinkie nail, a few grains of rice, or a quarter teaspoon of something. This gives your child the opportunity to see the food, touch it, smell it, and become more comfortable with it—with the idea that they will eventually be willing to try it. You could also put the small amount of food on a spoon, and if they don't taste it themselves, you can eat it. They'll never be able to try a food if it's not offered, and many kids are more likely to try something if it's there on their plate. So keep serving these foods and enjoying them yourself. One day, your child will come around.

Also think about how you're talking to your child about their eating. If they internalize the idea that they are a "picky eater," it becomes part of their identity, and the behavior becomes harder for them to change. They essentially "give up" on learning to eat new foods. To help your child avoid internalizing this label, avoid calling them a *picky eater*. Instead, use low-pressure phrases that encourage them to try the new food like, "You can eat it when you're ready," "You can try it a different time, " "You're learning to like it," and "You haven't learned to like it yet."

BE A FOOD MARKETER

Food companies aren't the only ones who can use fun and novelty to "market" foods to your child. So can you! Making family meals playful and fun can be a great way to engage your child in eating. One of my favorite food "marketing" strategies is a very simple one that I call *toothpick magic*. It involves cutting up your child's food into bite-size pieces and sticking a toothpick in each. That's it! I've seen my own (and other people's) kids try things I never thought they would thanks to toothpick magic. It works with adults, too!

Other ways to add fun to mealtimes might be to pretend you are a dinosaur eating "leaves" (lettuce), eating with a serving utensil just to be silly, or serving a meal on a cutting board or in a muffin tin for a different experience. You might also let your child help prepare foods in a more grown-up way—based on their readiness, you could teach them to use the peeler or how to use a knife.

In my house, we like to "taste test" foods that come in a variety of different colors, like apples, tomatoes, or bell peppers. We all compare the tastes of the different colors and vote on which we like best. One night when our family was doing this with bell peppers (red, orange, yellow, and green), the kids had the idea of turning it into a guessing game. One person would close their eyes and open their mouth, and another person would give them one of the bell pepper slices. Then the person with their eyes closed would try to guess which color they were eating. It was a lot of fun, even for the adults, and the kids each ate a whole bell pepper in the process. This is a great activity for kids of all ages, toddlers to teens.

IF THEY WON'T EAT THIS, SERVE THAT

You don't have to get wrapped up in your child's picky eating. You can play it cool, pretending that you don't care whether they try the new food or not. If Gemma, for example, is unwilling to eat one type of food, her parents could see if there is another food that is nutritionally similar that they can sub in at future meals.

Vegetables are important. It's also possible that your child will go through a phase where they won't eat many vegetables, but they will still eat fruit. If this is the case, serve fruit, which is also nutritious and has many of the same nutrients as vegetables (just don't give up on exposing them to vegetables!). Your child can take a short break from eating most vegetables and still be healthy.

If your child won't eat chicken or other meat and you wish they would, serve alternative protein sources like beans, eggs, nuts and seeds, nut butter and seed butter, tofu, and dairy. Sometimes for kids, the issue with meat is texture. These other protein-rich foods are easier to chew, and they have many of the same nutrients as meat (plus some others of their own). Your child can be a vegetarian and be healthy (be sure to read about supplements in chapter 5 if your child doesn't eat any animal products). Offer protein-rich foods at all meals and snacks.

REWARD WITH PRAISE OR WITH NONFOOD REWARDS

This may be effective for children who are:

- on the younger side (approximately six or under, but will vary by child)
- motivated by praise or rewards
- have a hard time trying foods a second time

This may be riskier for children who are:

- sensitive to praise being used to "get" them to do something
- already making progress with picky eating

Some kids have no desire whatsoever to try new foods, or else trying the new food is just a big hurdle for them to get over. Offering praise and nonfood rewards can motivate some of those kids to learn to try new foods. But keep in mind that rewards can also decrease a child's internal desire to try foods and learn to eat new foods on their own, because they start to rely on the reward. To reduce that risk, reward the action, not the child. Your child should know that they are a wonderful, lovable child regardless of whether or not they try a new food or eat a certain amount. This sounds like:

"Great job trying a new food. Here's your sticker!"

"You're taking a bite of that new food and earning five minutes of video game time!"

"Let's celebrate with a trip to the dollar store! You tried five new foods this week!"

It does not sound like:

"You're such a good girl for eating your veggies tonight."

If you decide to go this route, avoid using dessert or other desirable foods as the reward. Food incentives are one of the few things that child feeding researchers agree on, and they almost always observe the same thing: Kids who are incentivized with foods tend to be pickier and less able to listen to their hunger and fullness cues. So whenever possible, stick with nonfood rewards: stickers, small toys, high fives, calls to a relative, special privileges (like staying up five minutes later), or something else that is motivating for the child.

Remember, even when giving rewards for trying new foods, make it a point to follow as many of the practices of embodied independence (chapter 2) as you can. One risk to rewards is that it will override the internal signals a child gets from their body, so to help your child maintain their embodiment, you can make sure you are allowing them to choose how much to eat as often as possible within their constraints. You can also offer food options that work within your framework, like allowing your child to choose between two meal options or to choose what to eat for snack.

Finally, have an exit plan. Offering rewards for trying new foods doesn't have to be a forever strategy. Once your child is routinely trying new foods, you can start scaling back on rewards, which will allow them to gradually develop their own intrinsic motivation for trying new foods. For example, you could let your child watch a show if they try a new food. Then after they do that a few times, you could let them watch a show if they try a new food two days in a row. Then after they do that a few times, you could go to one show if they do it three days in a row, and so on.

Once they are routinely trying new foods on their own, you can stop the incentives.

WATCH FOR SIGNS OF MORE SERIOUS PICKY EATING

For some children, typical picky eating can get worse and veer into a more serious form of picky eating. Be aware of the following warning signs: If your child has an increasingly small list of foods they will eat; if they refuse to *ever* try a new food; if they are never willing to add a food back onto the list of foods they like; or if the picky eating disrupts family or social life, or a child's health. A few other red flags for eating problems include a family history of eating disorders or severely disordered eating, feeding problems as a baby or with solid food introduction, avoiding all foods of a certain sensory experience (like all wet foods), or refusing to eat an entire food group. If you are seeing any of these signs, your family may benefit from learning specific skills to prevent or manage extreme picky eating, covered in the next chapter. If your child is showing signs of nutrition problems or other health problems, checking in with their healthcare provider is important.

HIGH-RISK STRATEGIES TO AVOID

Force-feeding, "starving out," and punishment are not feeding strategies that I ever recommend for trying to get picky eaters to eat. Even when well intentioned, these methods are very risky, and it's difficult or impossible to reduce the risks.

Force-feeding, which involves activities like physically putting food into a child's mouth, holding their nose so that they will swallow, or using verbal threats or manipulation to get them to eat can sometimes happen when a parent is concerned that their child is not eating enough to meet their nutritional needs. "Starving a child out" involves providing only the foods you want your child to learn to eat and withholding all other foods until they are willing to eat the new or rejected foods—even if this means they are skipping meals. Punishing a child for not eating, whether it's sending them to their room, taking away screen time, or withholding dessert, can be problematic. Not only do punishments often exacerbate picky eating and make it last longer, but they can be traumatic for kids and may lead to a child having less respect for their body or their hunger and fullness cues.

APPLYING THE SIX-STEP FRAMEWORK FOR GEMMA

Returning to Gemma's story from the start of this chapter, let's consider how her parents might use the six-step framework to problem-solve for her feeding dilemma.

Step 1: Separate fact from fiction. Gemma's parents had started to tell themselves that withholding her favorite crackers when she refused a meal would *ruin* her relationship with food permanently. Another story they were telling themselves was that she would be a picky eater *for the rest of her life* if they couldn't convince her to eat a variety of foods now. After discussing the issue, they realized that they were imagining worst-case scenarios about Gemma's future eating habits that may never come to pass. Instead of worrying about the future, they decided to commit to doing what they could to improve her eating routine in the here and now.

Step 2: Pick the priority. Gemma's parents considered their relationship with each other, which was being strained by their disagreement over how to deal with her pickiness. They also made a list of their priorities, which included Gemma's embodied independence, Gemma's nutrition needs, and their schedules. They chose supporting their daughter's embodied independence as their number one priority.

Step 3: Brainstorm—with a twist. Next, her parents made a list of things they might experiment with to get her to try new foods, from the practical to the silly (What *would* happen if they put a mini fridge of vegetable pouches in her bedroom so she could eat them whenever she was hungry?).

Step 4: Take a risk reduction approach. After deciding to move forward with taking charge of the menu in the house and not offering Gemma's preferred snacks if she didn't eat the meal, her parents made a list of risk reduction strategies. They were concerned that not allowing her to respond to her hunger after meals would reduce her embodiment, so they decided to offer a "boring" snack if she did ask for food. They wished that the family could eat together every night, but since that didn't work for their schedules, they decided to have dinner together whenever they could to model good eating habits.

Step 5: Think like a scientist and start an experiment. They began to implement their plan. If Gemma didn't eat a meal or snack during the day, they would offer a small amount of one of the fruits or veggies she generally liked. They decided that if Gemma refused to eat the dinner that they offered, they would have a nutritious snack available for midnight wake-ups (some cheddar cheese slices), and they offered her substantial breakfasts that she could fill up on if she chose to. Additionally, they started eating dinner as a family three nights a week and eating the foods they wanted her to learn to eat again. They also started to praise her every time she tried a new food. They decided to reassess the situation in two weeks.

Step 6: Celebrate your wins, then continue to tweak your experiment. Gemma's parents congratulated themselves for getting on the same page regarding how to handle their daughter's pickiness. On the first day that they didn't give Gemma the crackers, she had a royal forty-five-minute tantrum, but they maintained a united front. After the smoke cleared, they made it through the meal, got Gemma down for bed, and gave each other a high five for sticking it out. After two weeks of their new approach, Gemma's parents noticed that she adored their praise and seemed willing to try new foods only when they praised her—she even waited to eat foods in general until they looked like they were watching and would give positive feedback. She was also having fewer tantrums when she didn't get crackers, and she was refusing dinner less.

The parents weren't comfortable with how their praise was

making Gemma less motivated to eat on her own, so they stopped praise entirely and decided to try being food marketers instead. They started putting Elmo stickers on bananas and oranges and packages of foods they wanted Gemma to eat. They added two family lunches and one family breakfast to their weekend schedules and focused family meals on making the meals fun and "playing" with the foods she was learning to like.

Gemma didn't magically become an adventurous eater, but she continued to eat a variety of foods from all the food groups, and she occasionally added some new foods to the list of what she would eat. She also sometimes stopped eating her favorite foods with no notice (which drove her parents bonkers). Her parents decided they would continue with their current plan for a while and keep an eye on whether Gemma's picky eating seemed to be getting better or worse.

11

EXTREME PICKY EATING AND ARFID

Typical picky eating is common, and with some intentional actions to avoid making it worse, it often resolves quickly. At the same time, picky eating can be the first signal that a child is at risk for more serious eating challenges. This chapter is all about those challenges—when picky eating progresses into something more, or when pickiness has been super serious from the get-go.

> "I've done all the right things, and they just aren't working. When my son was a baby, he ate everything, and slowly, he stopped eating anything. He hasn't tried anything new in three years. He's down to seven foods. I'm so defeated. I don't know what to feed him. Trying to go anywhere is a nightmare."

> "I had to drive all over the area for four hours to find a loaf of the one brand of bread my child will eat."

> "She really wants to go to camp, but she knows she can't because she wouldn't be able to eat there."

These are a sampling of the kinds of messages I get from parents struggling with extreme picky eating in their kids. They might be similar to something you've said, without even realizing that your kid's picky eating qualified as "extreme." Behaviors associated with extreme picky eating extend beyond the typical pickiness outlined in the previous chapter. Extreme picky eating is picky eating that interferes with a child's mental or physical health or social function, it has many risks, and it can be part of the serious clinical eating disorder ARFID (avoidant/restrictive food intake disorder). Extreme picky eating and ARFID are much bigger health concerns than typical picky eating. They can be disruptive to a child's health, growth, and social development, and they often are a source of major strain on a family. For parents who are wondering if their child's eating is aligned with indicators for ARFID or extreme picky eating, the Pediatric Screener for ARFID and Extreme Picky Eating (PSA-Eat) is a tool that can provide more information.

The classic recommendation for typical picky eating, which says you should keep exposing kids to new foods and they will learn to like them, will never be enough for extreme picky eating. Some kids do eventually outgrow extreme picky eating, but the longer they have it and more extreme it is, the more likely they will continue to be picky into adulthood with nutritional and social challenges. But even in these complicated cases, there are strategies that can move the needle in a positive direction for many kids.

Sam

Sam is a neurodivergent eight-year-old. He started out eating a lot of foods as a baby, but as he's gotten older, he has dropped foods from the list he is willing to eat to the point where now he eats only ten foods: one brand of frozen star-shaped chicken nuggets, boxed macaroni and cheese, milk, french fries from one fast-food restaurant, crackers, peanut butter, packaged mini muffins, carrots, dried apples, and chocolate candy. His parents worry about his health constantly. They think he is just being stubborn about trying new things and that his eating reflects their parenting skills. He was recently diagnosed with iron-deficiency anemia and routinely experiences painful constipation. When he goes to birthday parties, he brings his own food. Sam's parents are finding social situations increasingly difficult, and to be able to travel they need to pack all of his food and have a place to prepare it. In other areas of his life, Sam is generally doing well. He's on grade level at school, has friends, and likes to play soccer and do puzzles.

WHAT'S GOING ON?

There are a few factors that may be complicating your child's picky eating that your child doesn't have control over. To start, children with more "difficult temperaments" and negative emotions may be more likely to be severely picky. At the same time, it's my observation that most picky kids are, at least according to their parents, "stubborn." Far from the character deficit that some parents think it is, I think these kids are just insistent on protecting their bodies from uncomfortable experiences.

Some neurodivergent children or children with complicated eating also have a hard time with executive functions—all those skills that help people manage everyday tasks. Executive functioning skills include the ability to stay calm, flexible, organized, and more. These kids may struggle with flexibility. Food is the ultimate in unpredictability. Think about a bowl full of blueberries. One berry may be crisp and sweet. The next one may be hard and tart. Another one could be mushy and overripe. I have the skills to be flexible, so if I get a sour blueberry, I know it's just part of playing the blueberry lottery. If a child is inflexible, however, eating blueberries is a nightmare. This is why kids with extreme pickiness often prefer processed "white" or "beige" foods, such as cookies, cheese, breads, or pasta. They know what they will get every single time.

The most extreme form of picky eating is ARFID. ARFID has

several subtypes. In the anxiety subtype, a child may be very afraid of certain foods, afraid of choking or vomiting, or afraid of something else bad happening, so they don't eat. They may also have a complete lack of appetite. Having sensory sensitivities and difficulties processing sensory information is also a subtype of ARFID. Sensory processing refers to how a person's body handles the information it gets from their eight senses: sight, smell, touch, taste, hearing, balance, body awareness, and internal feelings. Some children experience these sensations in a way that makes it difficult for them to be able to eat, and they eliminate foods that have a certain sensory profile, such as only being able to eat dry, crunchy foods.

While we don't fully understand the causes of ARFID and extreme picky eating, a few of the risk factors include family history, difficulty feeding in early childhood, and being picky for a long time. Kids with neurodivergence, such as those with ADHD or autism spectrum disorder (ASD), are also likely at higher risk for extreme picky eating and ARFID, along with other eating challenges like low interoception and impulsivity, all of which make honoring body cues difficult. These conditions can result in poor growth, severely limited nutritional intake and food variety (increasing their risk of diseases like scurvy—from vitamin C deficiency), long-term picky eating, low bone density, and heart problems. It can also result in the child being underweight, which can be more serious than it sounds because it can make long-term recovery from ARFID much more difficult. Their picky eating often causes emotional turmoil for parents, mealtime conflict, and social challenges and isolation, such as not being able to travel or eat at and attend social events.

As eating disorders, ARFID and extreme picky eating are often treated from several angles. The first line of treatment is usually addressing a child's medical problems with their healthcare provider, which begins with regaining weight if needed (in serious cases, this could require tube feeding or hospitalization), followed by education for families on lifestyle strategies and techniques to support their child (sometimes called *family behavioral interventions*). Children with ARFID or extreme picky eating usually need techniques that develop their sensory processing skills, executive functions, and anxiety tolerance. These can be learned in family behavioral interventions, as well as one-on-one with specialists, such as dietitians, occupational therapists, feeding therapists, or psychologists. In some cases, using therapeutic techniques at home in the early years can prevent progression to more extreme forms of picky eating, or even prevent picky eating from ever becoming extreme picky eating. I've seen this happen in my own home as well as in the homes of the families in my BetterBites programs. It's never too late, even if your child is a tween, but intervening early is ideal.

START WITH THE BASICS

When it comes to extreme picky eating and eating challenges, the lowest-risk option is to focus on the core practices from part 1 of the book. Approach your child with curiosity, let them stop eating when they're full (and don't pressure them to eat more), serve a variety of foods to increase their exposure, set your menu at the eating independence restaurant, delay introduction of hyper-palatable foods (as strictly as possible), model a varied diet and eat together, consider whether supplementation may be needed, and take a factual and neutral approach to foods. Preparing foods with high calorie density may be an important part of maintaining your child's weight as well.

These are all low-risk activities. I've observed them helping *many* families like Sam's, with neurodivergent children and children with eating challenges, especially when they are used with children under five years old. With that said, for families with an extreme picky eater, these practices are important, but alone, they usually aren't enough to help these eaters add foods to their list of acceptable options or regain weight.

PROBLEM-SOLVING STRATEGIES TO TRY

The strategies that I'm about to share will likely be a good fit for some kids and carry more risk for others. As you experiment, observe how each strategy is affecting your child and your family. And as always, remember to consider *who* your child is and *how* you implement the strategies that you try. Pay attention to your child's reaction, avoid "you" language or talking about body shape and size, and take your child's perspective seriously.

EXPLAIN THE NEED TO EAT FOR HEALTH

This may be effective for children who are:

- curious or analytical
- need to know *why* before they do something
- motivated by information or like to know how their bodies work
- old enough to understand health information

This may be riskier for children with:

- obsessions with "good food / bad food" or disordered eating
- shame around their picky eating
- complete inability to try new foods
- insufficient language skills

Some kids respond well to hearing the *why* behind what you're asking them to do. For these kids, understanding what's going on in their bodies can be especially helpful. When they understand that their bodies aren't getting something nutritionally that they need, they may be more likely to try to eat that thing. Sam's parents, for example, might connect the dots between a particular food and helping with his constipation. You might do the same with something that's meaningful to your child, such as sports, activities, avoiding illnesses, building muscle, or not having to take a supplement that they do not like taking. When you are explaining what is happening in their body, throw in phrases like, "This is very common," "This happens to lots of kids," or "This happens to me, too, sometimes." These phrases will help your child see that their picky eating is not a personal failure. The goal is not to make them feel guilt, shame, or fear—it's to give them motivation to take care of their body.

If you have the kind of child who doesn't like to be told what to do (who does, really?) and who will resist every demand you place on them, beware of presenting the information as any form of pressure or instruction. Instead, sprinkle simple facts over the course of days when it makes sense (they will know if you're "making up" a reason to talk about it, so look for genuine opportunities that arise—you'll find them). You might say, "You're getting stomachaches from being constipated," or "I got some whole wheat bread today at the store. It has a lot of fiber in it." But don't try to jam too much information into a single conversation. Provide it gradually and naturally, perhaps over the course of several days or weeks.

Once you've used this strategy for a little bit, pay attention to their questions and comments about food. Take special note of whether your child is becoming overly interested in what they're eating or if they're cutting out other foods because of information they've received. Also note how they are talking about their health and if they seem to be worried about it. Some risks involved with this "convincing" approach are that children may become more anxious that they'll get sick, or that it may lead them to be perfectionistic about their health or what foods they eat. If you're noticing that your child's relationship with their body or food is starting to be affected, you might consider using a different strategy.

If Sam's parents were to try this strategy, they might say:

> "Iron is something that our bodies need to get oxygen. When you don't have enough, you might feel more tired when you're

playing soccer. We just learned from your blood test that you have low iron. This happens to lots of kids. Right now, the foods you eat don't have much iron in them. It would be helpful to add a food that has iron if we can. Here are some foods that have a lot of iron. Which one do you think you would like to start learning to like?"

Or

"You mentioned being constipated. If our bodies don't have enough fiber and fluid, we can't poop. The things you eat right now don't have a lot of fiber, which is why you are getting stomachaches. This happens to lots of kids and sometimes happens to us, too. The doctor has asked us to add in foods that have fiber, which can be tricky. So let's just start exploring one that all of us could learn to like. Which one would you like to start with?"

ALLOW DISTRACTIONS WHILE EATING

This may be for children who are:

- regulated or calmed by screens
- losing weight or experiencing health problems due to insufficient food intake and eat more while distracted
- get bored while at the table and won't stay seated

This may be riskier for children:

- who can't eat or get too distracted while watching screens or having other distractions
- who never, ever try new foods

For some kids, having distractions while eating can enable them to eat more foods and eat a wider variety of foods. It distracts them from the uncomfortable parts of eating so that they can continue. For others, it can help them regulate themselves enough to calmly eat a meal.

On the other hand, there are some kids for whom eating in front of screens can contribute to eating problems, maintain picky eating, or, in extreme cases, lead to kids being reliant on screens for the ability to eat. To reduce possible risks while using distractions, start with the least distracting distraction. Reading books or playing with toys can be a distraction that works for some kids, but that is less distracting than a screen. Some shows also may be less distracting than others. Reruns of old shows like *Mister Rogers* or slow nature documentaries may be a better fit than a nail-biter episode of their favorite cartoon that takes all their attention. And remember, it's harder to take things away than it is to add them. So start slowly. Instead of having distractions with all meals or snacks, begin with just one. See how it goes and if you can build skills they need during other meals and snacks.

Keep in mind that if your child is prone to eating past fullness, distractions can make it more difficult for them to observe their fullness cues. If that's true for your child, give them smaller starting portions and let them ask for more if they are still hungry. If you notice they are getting hungry before the next meal or snack, give them larger portions.

Ultimately, it would be great if your child could learn to eat without a screen or distraction, but if they are using distractions to regulate their emotions, you may need to teach them other regulation skills before you can take the screens away; things like breathing exercises, giving a child tight hugs or squeezes, altering the temperature or smells in the room, or increasing their oral stimulation with ice cubes or ice water could all work. If your child needs to be distracted from the sensations of eating, begin to expose them to food-related sensations outside of mealtime, such as having them help with grocery shopping or with some elements of food preparation. Once your child can better tolerate the eating experience, slowly begin to wean them off the distractions.

SET FIRM BOUNDARIES AROUND WHEN FOOD IS AVAILABLE TO MANAGE HUNGER AND FULLNESS CUES

This may be for children:*

- with executive function difficulties such as low impulse control

This may be riskier for children:

- with food insecurity or food trauma
- with high interest in "good foods / bad foods," guilt, or shame related to eating
- who are sneaking foods because they are being overly restricted
- who are not getting enough calories (even if it seems like they should be getting enough)

Hunger and fullness cues are essential if a child is struggling with ARFID or extreme picky eating. Without hunger, often picky eating symptoms are much worse. For children with executive function challenges, standard boundary approaches may not work. A standard boundary may look like telling your child to come back to the table or that the kitchen is closed. It could also include standing in front of the cabinet door if they are trying to grab a bag of cookies five minutes before dinner starts. A firm boundary, on the other hand, might look like keeping the food out of reach of a child, storing food in a place a child doesn't know about, or having a lock on the cabinet. These boundaries can help

---

* Firm boundaries may be recommended as part of eating disorder therapy and genetic appetite disorders. Treatment of those disorders is best handled with a team of healthcare professionals who can advise on the best interventions for your child. They will not be discussed in this section.

your child get used to eating on a routine, which activates their biological rhythm (including hunger and digestion), which can help them eat better. These boundaries may prevent your child from eating foods that are crowding out the nutrients they need to resolve their nutrient deficiencies or fuel their growth and health. They may also help them tolerate or even enjoy foods that aren't hyperpalatable. (If you do this, please keep in mind the strategies for doing so appropriately, like avoiding "you" language and grouping multiple foods together, which are outlined in chapter 12.)

SERVE MOSTLY HYPERPALATABLE FOODS

This may be for children:

- with dangerously low appetite
- who need to regain weight to the level that they can psychologically recover from ARFID

This may be riskier for children:

- with nutrient deficiencies or medical problems
- who have chronic GI problems such as constipation

Nourishment is a big focus for many children with ARFID. The importance of weight regain and stabilization cannot be understated. It is essential to their growth, but it also reduces their risk of relapse in the future. Tier 1 of the Health Impact Tiers is the most important in ARFID—specifically *calories*. Often parents balk when healthcare providers recommend milkshakes or potato chips for children with weight-gain issues, and obviously, we want to establish weight regain with as few hyperpalatable foods as possible. But the more serious the child's ARFID, often the less likely they are to eat normal food, and hyperpalatable food may be essential for their weight regain. Weight regain in this case is much more important than anything else (unless there is a competing medical issue). A child is much more likely to have full recovery if they fully regain weight, regardless of how the weight was gained.

HIGH-RISK STRATEGIES TO AVOID

Force-feeding, "starving out," and punishing are very high-risk options for dealing with extreme picky eating, and I do not recommend any of them, as it is difficult or impossible to reduce the risks.

Force-feeding can happen at home or in the feeding therapy setting (although that is becoming less common). I've heard parents share experiences of their child ending up in the hospital because of dehydration or malnutrition when they followed the advice of a medical professional that recommended starving out their extreme picky eater. These strategies are not safe for extreme picky eaters. And for kids with eating challenges, adding punishment to eating is not going to make eating an enjoyable experience that builds connection for the family.

APPLYING THE SIX-STEP FRAMEWORK FOR SAM

Step 1: Separate fact from fiction. Given the stress of the situation, Sam's parents are increasingly frustrated and exhausted. It's very easy to see Sam's behavior as intentional. His parents oscillate between anger, frustration, and worry about his health and weight, concerned that what he is doing will affect his permanent development over the course of his life. They decide to set aside their big-picture worries and the story that Sam is just being stubborn, and focus on the facts. They have a problem now, and Sam needs to eat better.

Step 2: Pick the priority. Sam's parents list their priorities: supporting Sam's nutrition and health, supporting his sensory processing skills, navigating the family's social challenges, and managing their own stress. They decide that the most important issue is his health and addressing Sam's iron deficiency.

Step 3: Brainstorm—with a twist. They take a minute to write down their options, even the "bad" ones. They jot down: meeting with Sam's doctor, having assessments performed, punishing Sam for not eating, letting him just survive on supplement drinks, letting him eat in front of screens, changing his diet, and more.

Step 4: Take a risk reduction approach. Sam's parents know that Sam doesn't respond well to demands, so trying to convince him to get on board won't work. Instead, they'll need to come up with a way to present the information that he will be able to accept. They also plan to offer Sam incentives for eating the iron-rich foods that he needs, along with a strategy for weaning Sam off these rewards over time.

Step 5: Think like a scientist and start an experiment. Sam's parents work with his doctor to determine the iron supplement dose he needs to be able to start to resolve his deficiency. They try several varieties before finding one that he is able to take. They also decide to get Sam evaluated by a pediatric occupational therapist. There is a three-to-six-month wait for the evaluation, but they begin a digital family education program right away to start learning therapeutic strategies, and work on his anxiety and executive function to help him try new foods.

Since Sam is very independent and doesn't respond well to demands, his parents don't tell him to eat new foods with iron, but they do begin to drop little bits of information here and there to help him learn about his body. They also start having him eat in front of a screen. Finally, they realize that he is very responsive to being incentivized to try new foods. They develop a plan to use video game time as a reward and then to slowly wean off the video games to allow Sam to develop intrinsic motivation. Sam's parents decide to reassess their plan in two weeks.

Step 6: Celebrate your wins, then continue to tweak your

experiment. Sam's parents are relieved that he is taking his iron supplement, and they take a moment to feel hopeful due to everything they are doing. In two weeks, they reassess. They realize he eats even less when watching a screen, so they decide to remove screens from mealtime. They continue with the other actions, though, which seemed to be working well, and they make a plan to reassess their strategy in a month.

12

WHEN A CHILD IS OBSESSED WITH SWEETS, CAN'T STOP EATING HYPERPALATABLE FOODS, OR IS SNEAKING FOOD

The previous four chapters in this section addressed the continuum of feeding—how to handle dilemmas as you get your child used to eating food and enjoying mealtimes as they age. But equally troubling for many parents is dealing with a child's *relationship* with food—whether that's an obsession with sweets or hyperpalatable foods, as we'll discuss here, or body-image focus that creates a negative or loaded relationship with certain foods. A fixation on sweets, in particular, is something I hear from parents a lot. One mom sent me the following message: "I have three kids, ages four, six, and eight. We've always had a small number of sweets, and it's been no big deal for the four- and six-year-olds. The eight-year-old, though, is obsessed with sweets, and food in general. He loves to eat! Anything, really. He loves vegetables, fruits, dinner foods, and sweets and snacks. We've done the same thing for all the kids, so I don't understand why he's so obsessed."

It can be confusing and concerning if your child sneaks food or is obsessed with sweets or any other food. If you have more than one child, you may have the same rules and limits (or no rules or limits) for all of them, and yet one may sneak and hide food while the others don't. There are often a lot of emotions involved in this situation for parents. First off, let me be clear: If your child is sneaking food, is obsessed with food, or can't stop eating, it is not a moral failing on your part or their part. I know that a lot of people judge these behaviors or blame the parents (too much restriction, not enough parenting, and so on). But I don't, and I don't think you should either. I do think these are behaviors to get curious about, however, because they may give you insight into your child and which strategies you're using that may need to change.

Leo

Four-year-old Leo has been sneaking sugary foods for the past three months. And not just sneaking them—obsessively sneaking them. If there are cookies or candy in the kitchen, he will grab them and hide under the table or in the closet to eat them. His parents have a balanced perspective on food and never stigmatized sweets as bad foods. They don't talk negatively about foods, and they give Leo routine access to sweets. Still, the number of sweets that Leo has been eating has gotten to the point where they are concerned about his health. They did not want to completely restrict him from having sweets, so they started hiding anything sweet that they brought into the house. Now, every day, Leo searches the house obsessively trying to find sweets. His parents have decided to bring up this concern with Leo's healthcare provider for advice.

WHAT'S GOING ON?

Popular opinion would have us believe that restriction is the only, or main, cause of food obsession or sneaking. The voices making this claim, however, are often exclusively working with adults who have disordered eating, not with kids. As we've discussed in chapter 2, restriction does not cause reactance or obsession with food in all kids, and reducing control over food may not decrease food sneaking. While restriction may contribute to sneaking in some cases, we are likely missing much more important factors if we focus on it.

Kids can be obsessed with hyperpalatable foods, eat large amounts of food, and sneak food for a variety of reasons, including a lack of impulse control, an innate love of food, or not getting enough calories or nutrition. If a child isn't getting what they need, they may be driven by their body to find the fastest source of calories, which is something sugary or processed. This isn't usually due to anything intentional on the parents' part. For example, parents may have started to opt for low-calorie or low-fat foods or cooking methods and inadvertently reduced how many calories their child is getting. The child could also be lacking protein and fat in their diet, which could make them "constantly hungry." If they are primarily eating sweets and simple carbohydrates like white bread and crackers without protein and fat, their blood sugar may be going up and down quickly instead of staying somewhat steady, which can also make some kids hungry.

Some kids who sneak food have a poor sense of interoception and simply can't tell when they are full. Also, if a child has experienced food insecurity, they might be motivated to stash food whenever it's available. This may last many years or a lifetime. I've met plenty of adults who experienced food insecurity as kids and still need to have a stock of food at home to feel food secure.

Sneaking food can also occur if a child feels guilt or shame surrounding the foods they want to eat. If a parent sets limits on foods using qualifications ("You can only have two cookies; *otherwise, it will be too many for you*") or foods are being constantly evaluated as good or bad ("It's not good to have too many unhealthy foods like cookies"), a child may feel ashamed about wanting to eat sweets or hyperpalatable foods. Sneaking food is a core behavior of many eating disorders, including binge eating disorder and bulimia nervosa. Food preferences and cravings may also be related to an imbalance in gut microbes, which may contribute to sneaking. For example, antibiotics may upset the gut balance, and if a child has recently been on antibiotics, it's possible they may crave sweets or simple carbohydrates.

In addition to all these potential factors, sneaking food could just be an issue of genetics, temperament, or something entirely unrelated to the food itself (one mom told me her kids snuck food because they really wanted to eat in their bedrooms). Clearly, there is no single thing "going on" here.

START WITH THE BASICS

CURIOSITY

When one of my kids was five, I noticed he was sneaking food first thing in the morning. So I got curious. Why was he sneaking food? He always has enough food, and we didn't stigmatize or overly restrict any foods. He was obviously hungry first thing in the morning, and after some thought, I guessed that he was looking for more independence with eating. So we put some food in a little section of the fridge for him to take out and eat on his own in the morning, and it solved the sneaking.

If your child is sneaking, be curious with them in a non-shaming way. Ask questions, warmly, and try to spot clues as to why they might be sneaking foods. *Warmly* is the key here, because the *how* of these words will make a difference. These conversations will sound different based on your child's age and whether they are old enough to articulate how they feel or why they might be sneaking food. You might say something like, "Hey, buddy, I found this in your room. Were you hungry?" Or, "If you want some cookies, you can let me know any time. Cookies are delicious and fun to eat; you don't need to hide to eat them. Maybe I'll want cookies at the same time as you, and we can eat them together! Were you worried you would get in trouble?"

If you find your child sneaking food, you might say something like, "Hi, sweetie. Looks like you're having a snack. Let's go sit at the table." Or, "I noticed you hiding those bar wrappers outside. I'm not worried about the bars, but I wonder why the wrappers are hidden." Then you can ask them questions at the table or later when they aren't eating.

Your child's sneaking might just be their idea of being silly—if you think that's the case and they know you know and it's like a game, have a little fun with it! However, since you have likely set limits in your household on when and where food is eaten after reading part 1 of this book, you will need to hold those limits in this moment, even if you decide to reevaluate and change them later. Holding limits might sound like, "Looks like you're eating candy under the table. Come on out. Candy is delicious, I know. It's hard not to eat candy all day when it's so yummy! You can give those candies to me [remove the candy]. We'll have more tomorrow." Or, "I found some snacks under your bed. I know it's fun to eat snacks in your room. We eat our snacks in the kitchen, not in your bedroom. Please throw the empty wrappers in the garbage right now."

MAKE SURE THEY'RE GETTING THE NUTRITION THEY NEED

When parents tell me their child is sneaking food, they usually expect me to ask them if they are saying certain foods are good or bad or restricting sweets. But if I spoke to Leo's parents directly, my first question would be—and has always been—"Are they getting enough fat and protein?" They may just be hungry and need more calories. Full-fat products, meals cooked with oil or fat, and a solid dinner or bedtime snack with fat and protein can help kids get the energy they need and stay full longer. Fat and protein can also help keep a child's blood sugar stable, which may affect their feelings of hunger and fullness or their drive to eat hyperpalatable foods. In my experience, this has solved the problem for many families.

SPEAK NEUTRALLY ABOUT FOOD

Consider how you talk about food, because if a child is hiding, they may be concerned that they will get in trouble or be shamed for eating certain foods or certain amounts of foods. They may need you to speak about food factually and from a morally neutral position, without assigning morality to eating certain amounts of food (eating less is "good," so if they want to eat more, they are "bad"). They may also need you to cut out any qualifications surrounding food, such as "That's enough ice cream for you." Make sure you are communicating warmly and supportively when it comes to food and eating, make sure you are giving structured permission, and be careful not to discuss body sizes or shapes in front of your child, either positively or negatively.

STRUCTURED PERMISSION

If your child loves hyperpalatable foods (and most do) but never knows when to expect that they will be served, or if they are always given a very small amount of these foods, they may really want more of that experience. It may be a good time to think about the situation from your child's perspective and consider whether they are experiencing it as structured permission (structure and boundaries with warmth) or restriction.

EMBODIED INDEPENDENCE

Make sure you're not rewarding with food. Rewarding with food can complicate a child's ability to listen to their body, and it can put certain foods on a pedestal. Also, make sure your "restaurant" is open when your child is hungry. They may need another eating opportunity if they can't fill up enough at one meal or are hungry at different times than when food is being offered.

SEEK OUT PROFESSIONAL HELP

Sneaking food can be a symptom of an eating disorder. If you suspect your child's behavior is not influenced by the factors discussed above (or even if it is, but the eating behavior is extreme), if you have a gut feeling that something is off, or if you know your child's risk of disordered eating is higher due to family history or other health factors, it's important to contact a professional with training in eating disorders. Warning signs include sneaking, hoarding, or binge eating foods routinely; refusing to eat around other people; or a child who feels like they are out of control with their eating.

PROBLEM-SOLVING STRATEGIES TO TRY

The ideas below will be helpful for some children and riskier for others. Bring the practice of curiosity with you as you experiment with these strategies because they will affect kids so differently. The *who* and the *how*—*who* your child is and *how* you implement these strategies—may matter more than the strategies themselves.

GIVE THEM MORE ACCESS

If kids are feeling shame or restricted around food, giving them less structure and fewer limits may be helpful. This could include serving a hyperpalatable food more often or in larger quantities or allowing your child to choose the quantity of hyperpalatable food to eat at certain times.

This approach may be effective for children who:

- are feeling guilt or shame about eating
- are concerned about their body size or shape, or are showing signs of disordered eating
- have an increased risk for certain eating disorders
- are feeling overly restricted
- have a history with food insecurity or trauma

This approach may be riskier for children who:

- are neurodivergent with increased feelings of reward from hyperpalatable foods

- have poor interoception or eating regulation
- have poor gut health or health challenges
- are not sneaking because they are feeling deprived

If your child has experienced food insecurity or trauma, then offering 24-7 access to food, plus a consistent and reliable meal and snack routine, may be the best fit. This might include letting them keep some snacks in their bedroom, and/or making sure there is a snack drawer or cabinet in your kitchen that is stocked and available in between meals. Regardless of whether this increases their risk of eating more hyperpalatable foods, a sense of security about food is essential and should be prioritized.

Many parents have told me that, for them, this approach has resulted in their kids becoming *more* obsessed with sweets or other hyperpalatable foods, because the more they eat, the less they want to eat "normal" foods, which makes them eat more hyperpalatable foods, and they get into an unhelpful cycle. It can also reduce their overall nutrition status. If this is the case, consider reducing the novelty factor of these items. It's human nature to be more interested in new things, which is one reason food companies are constantly adding new and "limited edition" flavors to hyperpalatable foods. If your child is obsessed with a food, making it available more often wears out the novelty and eventually the food becomes "boring." Keep in mind, if your child has been obsessed with a certain food (or foods) and they suddenly have unlimited access, they may act even more obsessed with it for a few weeks. I recommend giving it a month or so before you decide whether you want to continue with this strategy.

Practically speaking, reducing the novelty of hyperpalatable foods involves keeping all foods on a level playing field. Hyping up sweets, rewarding with food, and making kids finish their plate to get dessert can make certain foods more interesting and feel more rewarding to their brains. To take foods off a pedestal, try serving a small child-size portion of dessert *with* a meal rather than as a reward for finishing the meal. For some kids, this is a game changer—it puts broccoli on the same level as ice cream (I find this is especially effective for younger kids). Also, avoid hype situations like, "Oh wow! You're so lucky you got all that candy for your birthday!" As always, as you give more access, stay curious about how your child is responding. After the first month of trying this strategy, if you find your child is ramping up and eating more hyperpalatable foods, or becoming even more obsessed with food the fewer restrictions they have and it's beginning to crowd out other foods from their diet or affect their health in a meaningful way, you may decide this isn't a good fit and consider what type of structured permission might be a better fit.

HOLD FIRM BOUNDARIES

Sometimes there are foods or amounts of foods that kids cannot have for specific reasons. In these cases, firm boundaries may be needed.

This approach may be effective for children who:*

- have a medical condition
- are not meeting their nutrient needs
- are having health problems because of their eating
- have executive function difficulties such as poor impulse control

This approach may be riskier for children with:

- increased risk of eating disorders
- feelings of shame or guilt about food, their bodies, or their appetite
- past food insecurity

---

* Firm boundaries may be recommended as part of eating disorder therapy and genetic appetite disorders. Treatment of those disorders is best handled with a team of healthcare professionals who can advise on the best interventions for your child. They will not be discussed in this section.

A firm boundary might look like putting food where a child cannot access it or locking the cabinet. Keep in mind, though, that having food locked can feel icky to some kids (and parents), may contribute to a sense of deprivation, and could lead to guilt and shame related to eating. (This is especially true of a child with any history of food insecurity, and I highly recommend against this strategy in that case.) For these reasons, consider using this strategy only with young kids.

When I had my second son, my first son learned the skill of opening the refrigerator door. He was two years old. Like most toddlers, he didn't have much impulse control. We put a lock on the refrigerator door. It kept everyone safe. Many young kids are used to having cabinets locked whether there are cleaning supplies, breakables, or choking hazards behind the door. It's with older kids that we begin to think about the risks and how these strategies may affect their relationship with their bodies or with food.

To help avoid a "good food / bad food" mentality, consider storing multiple types of foods together so that when you lock the cabinet, it's not just the hyperpalatable foods being singled out. If your child asks you why the cabinet is locked, you can say something like, "It's tricky to leave the cabinets closed when it's not snack time, so this makes it easy for us," rather than "You can't respect the rules, so we need to do this." Using *us* rather than *you* in your language avoids putting blame on your child.

If you are locking up food or making it otherwise unreachable, make sure that you provide a very predictable meal and snack schedule so that your child knows exactly when food will be available and that you are reasonable with how often the food is available. If you usually lock the snack drawer and make it available only once a week, that may not feel like enough from your child's perspective. If you want certain foods to only be available that infrequently, not purchasing the foods could be a better risk reduction strategy than your child knowing they are always in the house and almost always unavailable.

Because locking up food comes with real risks, I recommend using this strategy for as short a time as possible. In settings beyond the kitchen, start to teach your child about impulse control skills through such games as red light, green light; Simon says; or freeze tag. Once your child begins to develop more self-control skills, they may be able to follow the limits better. You can also teach eating regulation skills by helping develop your child's sense of interoception (see ideas in chapter 2). And if your child's health issue resolves, you can remove the firm boundaries.

MAKE A SHARED DECISION WITH YOUR CHILD

If you have a big kid, tween, or teen, involving them in the limit-setting process can be a key to getting them on board with a change. Whether you're increasing or decreasing their access, they likely have opinions about what they need or want.

This approach may be effective for children who:

- are old enough to come up with ideas, especially tweens and teens
- have some flexibility with their health status
- have disordered eating symptoms

This approach may be riskier for children who:

- are experiencing health problems because of their eating intake

When implementing this method, ask questions like, "What snacks would you like me to buy so that you always have something to eat?" "Would you like to have dessert more often?" or "We're going to have drinks other than soda now. Which sparkling waters should we try?" Of course, if you start this conversation, it's only fair to take your child's opinions and preferences seriously. That may mean serving dessert more than you'd prefer or buying foods that weren't your first choice. You will want to use this approach only if your child has some health flexibility and you are willing to take some of their preferences into account.

TAKE A BREAK FROM HYPERPALATABLE FOODS

In some cases, your child may be so used to eating hyperpalatable foods that they want to eat only hyperpalatable foods, and they stop eating normal food completely. Maybe nutrition went out the window during the holidays or you went through a busy season and ate only processed foods. If this is the case, their diet has gotten way out of balance, and they need a reset for their body and taste buds.

This approach may be effective for children who:

- have stopped eating most normal foods
- have a gut imbalance
- have a strong understanding that all foods are good and do not have morality attached to them
- have very unbalanced diets

This may be riskier for children with:

- extreme picky eating
- food insecurity or food trauma
- disordered eating symptoms or who are overly interested in which foods are "good or bad"

If you decide to try this approach with your child, keep in mind that taste buds regenerate pretty quickly—after about two weeks—which means that human taste preferences can adjust in about that amount of time. If you've been used to eating a high-sodium diet and then you eat a low-sodium diet, initially the food will taste bland. After about two weeks, though, your taste buds will change and you'll become used to the new level of sodium. If you go back to a high-sodium diet, it will initially taste way too salty.

Of course, taking a break from hyperpalatable foods is a hard sell for a kid obsessed with them, and there is the risk that for some kids it may contribute to an unhealthy mentality about food. For kids with extreme picky eating, it may lead to malnutrition if the child is not able to eat the alternative foods. For kids with a history of food insecurity, it could also trigger a sense of deprivation or trauma response. To reduce some of the risks associated with cutting out hyperpalatable foods, speak neutrally about the foods you are taking a break from. There's no need to explain that certain foods are "bad." For a younger child, you don't have to explain at all; you can just change their diet. For a big kid, you might say something like, "Our bodies need all kinds of foods. We've been eating so many sweets and salty snacks that we haven't had room for other foods. So we're going to take a break from those for a few weeks and try lots of the other foods we've been missing. We'll find out which ones we like." You could also say, "We've been eating a lot of sweet and salty foods. They're fun to eat, and also, we've gotten a little out of balance and our bodies have forgotten how to like foods that aren't sweet and salty. We're going to give our taste buds two weeks to regrow with less sugar and salt so that they learn to like other foods again, and then we'll add fun foods back in."

If you're asking the kids to take a break, make sure you're doing it, too. Let your child know that the whole family is in it together so that they won't feel unfairly singled out or like they are the problem. At the same time, if you're removing hyperpalatable meals from your child's diet, make sure you're going the extra mile to offer meals that taste good and are satisfying. Also, don't keep the foods you're taking a break from in the house—refrain from buying them altogether.

After taking a break, you might consider reintroducing some

of the hyperpalatable foods. Whether you take an unlimited approach or a structured permission approach, it will be important for your child to understand that you can enjoy hyperpalatable foods and be healthy.

HIGH-RISK STRATEGIES TO AVOID

The following actions are very risky, and I would not recommend them, as it's difficult or impossible to reduce the risks.

CONSISTENTLY IGNORING THE BEHAVIOR

If your child snuck foods once or twice or went through a phase when they were obsessed with food and then it stopped, that's one thing. (In the latter case, it may have been a growth spurt.) If your child, however, is consistently sneaking or if they are obsessed with food and it's impacting their life, then it needs to be addressed.

PUNISHING THEM TO GET THE BEHAVIOR TO STOP

Something is pushing your child to eat in the way they are eating. Punishing them is not going to address the underlying reason, and it likely will not even stop their behavior. Taking away screen time because they snuck candy before dinner isn't going to address the fact that they were hungry before dinner and dinnertime needs to be moved up. If we're not addressing the reason, we're setting our whole family up for failure.

KEEPING AN IRON GRIP ON ALL FOOD LONG TERM

Except in rare circumstances like genetic disorders, being extremely restrictive will not give your child the tools they need to learn to listen to their body and have a good relationship with food. It could likely do the opposite—teaching them they cannot trust their body, that it's a moral failure to eat in certain ways, or pushing them to eat in a way that is even more hazardous to their health.

As your child gets older, they will naturally have and need more independence with eating and food choices.

APPLYING THE SIX-STEP FRAMEWORK FOR LEO

Step 1: Separate fact from fiction. Initially, Leo's parents were divided on what the "bigger story" was. Were they bad parents? Was Leo a rebellious child who didn't respect them? Was he going to sneak and binge on food for the rest of his life? Was this the beginning of a binge eating disorder? They decided they needed to take a step back and separate fact from fiction. The facts of the matter were that Leo was sneaking food and the parents were trying to stop it.

Step 2: Pick the priority. After considering several priorities, including supporting Leo's physical health, supporting his relationship with food and his body, and reinforcing appropriate behavior and respect toward his parents, Leo's parents decided to reach out to Leo's healthcare provider for help in choosing their top priority. Together, the parents and provider decided that the first course of action should be to make sure Leo was getting all the calories, fat, and protein he needed, as it might just be that he was hungry and they wanted to avoid poor nutrition.

Step 3: Brainstorm—with a twist. Leo's parents decided to consider several strategies they had never considered before, including taking a full break from sweets and offering Leo unlimited sweets. They also considered the ideas the healthcare provider provided and ended up with a list of options—many more than they thought they had, which felt freeing. They took a minute to discuss potential pros and cons of these strategies together and with their child's healthcare provider.

Step 4: Take a risk reduction approach. When consulted, Leo's healthcare provider asked many questions and noted that Leo had recently been on a short course of antibiotics, which affected his gut health, and that his parents had gotten into the habit of purchasing low-fat and nonfat foods and cooking lower-calorie meals for their own health. The healthcare provider also learned that Leo primarily sneaked sweets in the morning before breakfast and that there was some family history of disordered eating. As a group, they decided that the biggest risks to Leo right now were developing an eating disorder and becoming malnourished due to an imbalanced diet. So as they considered strategies, they looked for actions that would reduce that risk.

Step 5: Think like a scientist and start an experiment. Leo's parents added more fat to all his meals, made sure a protein food was available with all meals and snacks, and added a bedtime snack to their nighttime routine. They decided to keep their firm boundaries given their concerns about Leo's gut health, but they also decided to provide a child-size portion of dessert with dinner every night, so that Leo knew when he would get sweets every day. They also provided other opportunities for sweets as they came up, along with a balanced diet. This seemed like a strategy that would reduce his risk of increasing rigidity over food being either good or bad, while still protecting his health.

The parents continued to use neutral language and included all foods in Leo's diet. Now, if they caught him sneaking food, they worked on warmly saying something like, "Looks like you have some candy. I know it's really yummy and you want to have that now. We'll have some with dinner." They kept the risk of disordered eating in mind as they started this experiment, watching for continued sneaking, obsessions with candy, shame, or other symptoms.

Step 6: Celebrate your wins, then continue to tweak your experiment. Leo's parents were proud that they made some real changes, and they were especially happy to see that Leo responded quickly and stopped sneaking food. He continued to have a sweet tooth and remained a bit fixated on treats, so his parents decided to make a tweak and pivot to an unlimited approach to sweets, rather than having firm boundaries. He started eating more sweets than ever before, but his parents gave it some time, knowing that it might take a while for the novelty or reactance to wear off. At this point, his parents decided to take a moment to congratulate themselves again. They made a decision, they made a change, and now they were gathering the data. Whether this experiment was "working" or not, they could acknowledge their efforts and their commitment to the health of their family.

After six weeks, Leo was more obsessed and eating even more sweets than at the start of the experiment. Sweets started crowding out other foods, including the foods with fat and protein that Leo needed, so the parents took the data they got from the experiment and decided an unlimited approach wasn't right for him at this time. Next, they moved to a structured permission approach, tweaking their experiment. They continued to offer a small amount of dessert with dinner every night, and they made cookies and milk available for his afternoon snack twice a week. They also allowed him to have a piece of candy with his lunch on Saturday and Sunday if they had it in the house left over from a holiday or party.

Leo continued to be a bit obsessed with candy, and when he had opportunities, like at birthday parties, he usually overate it, but he wasn't showing any signs of guilt or shame related to how much he ate, nor did he start sneaking foods again. He also wasn't talking about food in healthy and unhealthy terms, and he showed no signs of voluntarily restricting himself. Although his parents wished Leo weren't obsessed with candy and that he were able to self-regulate in a way that made him feel good, they could see that he needed more skills before he would be able to do that in a way that also preserved his health. They continued with their structured permission experiment for now, focusing on remaining morally neutral about all foods, including sweets.

13

CONCERNS ABOUT BODY IMAGE AND DISORDERED EATING

I routinely hear from parents whose kids are struggling with their weight or body image, and their relationship with food is being damaged as a result:

> "My very thin daughter, who is seven, just told me she needs to lose weight."
>
> "My three-year-old niece told my dad (her grandfather) she couldn't have chocolate because it would make her fat."
>
> "My son is obsessed with building his abs, so he turns down treats like celebratory ice cream. He's nine!"
>
> "My child's friend put herself on a 1,300-calorie-per-day diet—the kids are twelve years old! That doesn't feel right."
>
> "My son told me his friends are making fun of him for being fat and he's so unhappy with his body."

I've heard similar stories from my own son. When he was in fifth grade, he told me about comments some of his friends were making about weight and other people's bodies. "They all say the most weightist things," he told me. We'd been discussing the idea of weightism (defined as stigma or bias against people who have a higher weight) for years, so I wasn't surprised that he noticed, but even I *was* surprised at just how often kids were saying these things. Conversations that stigmatize weight start early. The thin ideal is pervasive in our culture, putting a certain body type on a pedestal—one that is slim and smooth, or built and muscular with low body fat. You can try your hardest not to engage in weightist talk in your home (and it's worth it), but kids will still pick up on it when they are out in the world—at school, summer camp, birthday parties, friends' houses. Our children are growing up in diet culture, and sometimes we're struck speechless by what they tell us or ask us, yet we have to say something.

Lauren

Lauren is an eight-year-old who loves to ride her bike, draw, watch movies with her family, and connect with her friends at school. Some of her friends have started to eat only vegetables for lunch because they want to "stay thin," and one has started to count calories. Lauren has always had a higher weight than most kids her age, and recently, her healthcare provider told her parents—in front of her—that she was overweight. Last week, several of the boys at school teased Lauren for being "fat." After that happened, when she got home, she told her moms that she needed to lose weight.

WHAT'S GOING ON?

Weight stigma is everywhere. In chapter 2, we discussed the outside influences that perpetuate the thin ideal, weight stigma, and diet culture—it can come from media, food marketing, family members, and even the medical establishment. I also outlined the risk factors for eating disorders. This chapter will focus on how to talk to your child about these topics, and I'll offer ideas for navigating eating dilemmas related to disordered eating and body image struggles, as well as pointing out red flags that indicate professional help may be needed.

START WITH THE BASICS

EMBODIED INDEPENDENCE

Recently, I started a fitness program to build back some of my muscle after a sedentary season of life. At the beginning of the program, I couldn't do a push-up. After a few months of sticking with my workouts, though, I was able to do some push-ups and, one day, I noticed my biceps were bigger. The size of my arms doesn't mean much to me, but I was excited that the workouts were doing something and that I was getting stronger, so I went and showed off my new biceps to my family.

I got to thinking about it later. Was it helpful to show off my muscles to my two sons? I try to make it a point of not talking about my body in terms of weight or size, for the purpose of discouraging the "thin ideal" and disordered eating, as well as to promote body acceptance. I would never have said anything to my kids if the workouts had led to weight loss. As I thought back on how I'd talked to my kids about my workout gains, I realized that I would have been better off focusing on what I really care about—my increased health and strength. Instead of talking about the size of my muscles, I could have said things like: "I can carry this huge pot of water across the house now," "I was able to work in the yard the whole day without getting tired," "I can do fourteen push-ups because I've been sticking with this for the past seven months." Or, most important, "I can tie my eleven-year-old in a minutes-long squat contest and not be sore the next day!"

A mom once came to me with an honest inquiry: "How do I use neutral language when my kids ask me a question, if I don't feel neutral about it? I do worry about my kids' weight and size, because other kids can be cruel."

Kids *are* cruel. So are adults. A child experiencing weight stigma or bullying needs extra support—and extra tools—to be able to cope and avoid internalizing these messages. But if a child believes that their body (rather than the bully) is the problem, not only will they be more susceptible to the bullying, they will also have the added burden of believing that they should try to alter their body, whether that's something they can control or not. We need to help our kids have embodied independence, which includes working on our own internalized weight bias. If a parent on some level believes that their child's body is too big or needs to stay small, that could easily come through in a conversation, even if the parent doesn't say it explicitly. Kids need us to be on their team. If a parent is having a hard time accepting a child's body size, it may be helpful for them to think about their own relationship with their body and, if they are struggling, seek out support for themselves.

FACTUAL LANGUAGE

Just like it can be helpful to talk about food using facts instead of judgments, it can be helpful to talk about bodies in the same way. If you are working on decreasing internalized weight bias in yourself and your family, consider using adjectives like *round*, *curvy*, *soft*, *firm*, *smooth*, and *bumpy* when talking about bodies or body shape, rather than saying *flabby*, *chubby* (in some contexts), or *chunky*. Or try phrases like, "Muscle makes our bones move," "Fat keeps us warm, stores energy, and protects our organs," "Bodies come in all shapes and sizes," and "Calories are energy."

Whenever I give examples of speaking factually about bodies online, there are always people who jump in with comments like, "But I'm not going to lie to my child about obesity!" These commenters argue that weight is solely the result of poor lifestyle choices, and they insist on the importance of telling their kids about how extra weight is bad, and about how they need to eat a certain way to stay thin. They claim that speaking about fat in a neutral way is deceiving their children. It strikes me that these commenters are *so* defensive of their weight-focused perspectives and weight stigma, and I wonder about where it comes from.

I believe in the importance of teaching our kids to respect people of all shapes and sizes, without fixating on anyone's size, passing moral judgment on them as a person, or deciding that another person should be trying to change the size of their body without knowing anything about them. You can take your child's health and nutrition very seriously and teach them about taking care of their body without teaching them to judge people with bigger bodies.

Here's another dilemma that I encountered recently: A mother shared that she taught her son that calories were energy. She presented this to him in a factual way, explaining that we need energy to grow and play. Her son loved that idea and started to ask for more food than he usually ate, looking at the nutrition labels to see how many calories they had so that he could "get more energy." The mom wasn't sure what to say, because she didn't want to contribute to weight stigma or dieting mindset, but she also didn't want her son to ignore his fullness cues just because he thought he would have more energy. Here's the script I shared with her, which uses factual language:

"Your body has a certain amount of energy. Food gives you the energy you need, but not extra energy. If you want to have the most energy your body can have, you can go to bed on time, play and move around every day, eat foods from all the food groups, listen to your body when it says it is hungry and full, and spend time with family and friends. The numbers you see on the labels can't tell you what your body needs—only your body can tell you that. Labels aren't for kids."

I'm a fan of the facts. Your child's body size will change constantly as they grow. They need to understand that this is healthy and normal, and they also need to understand how their body works. And if something unhealthy is taking place, then it needs to be communicated carefully. By sticking to facts rather than judgments about body size, shape, and appearance, the hope is that we'll give our kids a positive way of taking care of their ever-changing bodies. As parents, we can do our part to counter the never-ending stream of judgmental body and diet talk that surrounds us.

STRATEGIES TO TRY

LISTEN, VALIDATE, ENGAGE (LOVE)

When your child comes to you with a tricky question or concern about their body, it's important to first *listen* and then *validate* their concern, no matter what it might be. Once you have listened and validated, they might also need you to *engage* with their concern to offer a solution or a new way to think about it. I like to throw in an *o* for fun and use the acronym LoVE as a reminder of the importance of this strategy. When Lauren approached her moms about wanting to diet, she needed them to *love* her in that moment, exactly as she was. When any of our kids bring up the trickiest of tricky questions or statements, they need the same. Here's a breakdown of the elements of this strategy:

Listen. Your child needs to feel heard, and you need to make sure you understand what they are saying and what the context is. Listening includes letting them talk; asking questions to make sure you understand their perspective, what happened, or why they are asking the question; and repeating back to them what you heard, perhaps adding something to the effect of, "Did I get that right?"

Validate. Your child needs to feel like you are on their side and that their feelings and concerns are valid (even if you disagree with them). Validating starts with telling your child that their emotions make sense, perhaps saying something like, "It makes sense that you're upset," "You're right, he had no right to say that," or, "I would feel that way, too." Don't immediately try to cheer your child up—be willing to embrace the discomfort of letting them be upset. Finally, if it's appropriate, connect with your child by sharing a story of something similar that happened to you, to show them that you can relate to their experience.

Engage. Your child needs your support to navigate body conversations. Some of this may happen in the moment, and some of it may happen later as a follow-up to the initial conversation. Engaging may mean responding with assurance that you love and support your child, sharing some factual information with them about bodies or food, or offering a different way of thinking about the situation and helping your child to brainstorm solutions.

The following scenarios exemplify LoVE in action:

If your child says, "I'm fat"

If your child is smaller, you might immediately want to jump in with "No, you're not!" If your child is smaller or bigger, your instinct might be to say, "You're perfect just the way you are!" The problem is, the first response reinforces the idea that fat is bad, and the second response invalidates your child's experience. Instead of jumping in immediately with a response, begin by trying to find out what your child means by this statement in a low-pressure way. Do they mean it descriptively and neutrally? Does "fat" mean something negative to them? Did someone say something hurtful to them, which has caused them to say this? Are they upset about their body? A conversation with a child who is larger could look like this:

Nine-year-old: "I'm fat."
Parent: "Why do you say that?"
Nine-year-old: "A boy called me fat during recess."
[*Parent learns there's a social component.*]
Parent: "What do you think he meant by that?"
Nine-year-old: "He was being mean." [*Parent learns the child is using fat as a negative descriptor.*]

Parent: "How did you feel when he said that?"
Nine-year-old: "I was mad. He's not allowed to talk about people's bodies." [*Parent learns the child may be more upset about him breaking the rules and being mean than about their own body.*]
Parent: "You're right. No one should talk about other people's bodies. It makes sense that you're mad. Thank you for telling me this; it's important for me to know."
Nine-year-old: "Can I play video games now?"
[*Afterward, the parent continues to reinforce the idea that it's not okay to talk about other people's bodies, and keeps an ear out to see if weight teasing is becoming a pattern.*]

Or it could also play out in another way:

Nine-year-old: "I'm fat."
Parent: "Why do you say that?"
Nine-year-old: "My tummy sticks out too far." [*Parent learns child is unhappy with their body.*]
Parent: "I can see your tummy is round. Mine is, too. Were people at school talking about tummies?"
Nine-year-old: "Yes. Mine stuck out the farthest, and everyone saw it." [*Parent learns there is a social comparison.*]
Parent: "I bet that was hard to be different from everyone else."
Nine-year-old: "I wish my tummy were smaller." [*Parent learns child wishes their body were different.*]
Parent: "Bodies come in all shapes and sizes. It's hurtful when people think some shapes are better than others."
Nine-year-old: "Yeah."
Parent: "I'm sorry that happened, sweetie. That's really hard."
Nine-year-old: "Yeah."
Parent: "Thank you for telling me this. . . . Do you want to see if we can finish that puzzle we've been working on?"

⟦*Afterward, parent looks for opportunities to ask the child what they like about themselves, as well as to find books from the library that positively feature rounder characters.*⟧

For a child who is thin, the conversation could go differently:

Nine-year-old: "I'm fat."
Parent: "Why do you say that?"
Nine-year-old: "See this?" ⟦*grabs some skin*⟧ ⟦*Parent still doesn't know the child's concerns.*⟧
Parent: "Well, what you're grabbing right now is actually skin with not much fat. Was someone talking about fat recently?"
Nine-year-old: "I dunno, but I don't want to have fat." ⟦*Parent learns the child is thinking about fat negatively.*⟧
Parent: "Did you hear somebody say something bad about fat?"
Nine-year-old: "My friends are skipping lunch because they don't want to be fat. I don't want to skip lunch." ⟦*Parent learns the child has been exposed to dieting.*⟧
Parent: "I can see how you wouldn't want to skip lunch. You don't want to be hungry!"
Nine-year-old: "Yeah."
Parent: "Bodies come in all shapes and sizes with different amounts of fat. All bodies are good. It's important for everyone, including your friends, to eat all their meals and not skip them no matter what their body shape is. That's how you have energy to play, learn, and grow."
Nine-year-old: "Okay." ⟦*They wander off.*⟧
⟦*Parent makes a mental note to occasionally talk about how it's important to always eat all meals—and snacks, too, if you're hungry—to reinforce the idea that we shouldn't be skipping meals.*⟧

If your child says, "I need to lose weight"

Just as in the example above, your first instinct might be to jump in with "No, you don't!" or "You look fine the way you are!" These statements, however, can add internalized weight bias or invalidate what your child is experiencing. When your child brings this up, it's important to figure out what they really mean. No child wants to lose weight for weight's sake. Potential reasons why a child may say they need to lose weight include: They're being bullied or teased, they're repeating what their friends have said or are worried about trying to fit in, they're feeling lonely or rejected by their peers, or they're worrying about their health after a medical visit or after exposure to health education. It could be a combination of these factors, as is the case for Lauren. You want to address their concern, not the fact that they want to diet. For a smaller child, a scenario could look like this:

Seven-year-old: "I need to lose weight."
Parent: "Why do you need to lose weight?"
Seven-year-old: "My friend said I did." [*Parent learns the child is repeating a friend.*]
Parent: "I wonder what they meant by that."
Seven-year-old: [*Child shrugs.*] [*Parent learns the child doesn't really know how to interpret the situation.*]
Parent: "Bodies come in all shapes and sizes, and you don't need to do anything. It's not okay that your friend was talking about your body."
Seven-year-old: "Okay."

For a larger child, a scenario could look like this:

Seven-year-old: "I need to lose weight."
Parent: "Why do you need to lose weight?"
Seven-year-old: "My friends said I did." [*Parent learns there is a social component.*]
Parent: "I wonder what they meant by that."

Seven-year-old: "They said I'm too fat and they aren't friends with fat kids." [*Parent learns the child is worried about being socially rejected.*]
Parent: "Ugh. I wonder how that felt."
Seven-year-old: "Bad."
Parent: "I'd feel that way, too. When I was eight, some kids said that to me, too. I felt so sad I had to go in from recess crying."
Seven-year-old: [*says nothing*]
Parent: "It's not okay to talk about people's bodies. And not okay that they said they wouldn't be your friend because of your shape. That was so mean."
Seven-year-old: [*says nothing, but seems relieved*]
[*Parent decides to actively look for families to spend time with who have children who may have experienced similar situations.*]

Your child has a healthcare appointment focused on weight or BMI

For children with high weight or BMI, weight is often the first (or only) thing healthcare providers want to discuss. One mom told me, "My thirteen-year-old son said he needed to start running to lose weight after his doctor told him his BMI was high." First, if you are concerned that this might happen at your child's next appointment (regardless of your child's weight), you can call ahead and tell the healthcare provider that you do not want them to explicitly discuss your child's weight. You can also ask for *blind weighing*, where they weigh the child with the child's back turned to the scale number, and then write the weight down without verbally sharing it. It's still important to discuss your child's health, however, and potentially their lifestyle as well, so be open to discussing those topics during appointments. If your child does have a stigmatizing experience at the doctor's office, even if they don't bring it up with you, it's important to address it.

Imagine you're at the doctor with your child, and the doctor says, in front of your child, "She's already overweight, and her BMI is trending off her curve. If you don't get a handle on this now, she'll become obese. You need to put her on a diet. Cut way back on her carbs."

Later, you want to address the comments with your child.

Parent: "That doctor made some comments about your weight today. How did you feel about them?"
Twelve-year-old: "Do I have to go on a diet?"
Parent: "I'm not going to put you on a diet. The doctor didn't even ask about how you eat right now. He just assumed you were not eating a balanced diet."
Twelve-year-old: "What's 'obese'? Am I going to become obese?"
Parent: "Obese means a larger body. Our bodies are always changing. We don't know how our sizes and shapes will change in the future, and that doctor doesn't know either. Our job is to take care of our bodies the way they are right now."
Twelve-year-old: [*silence*]
Parent: "What that doctor said was an example of weight bias, where a person assumes something about another person because of their weight. That's not okay."
Twelve-year-old: "No, not okay."

Following an experience like this one at your child's doctor's office, instead of putting your child on a weight-loss diet immediately, it would be more helpful to learn possible causes for a child unexpectedly gaining weight beyond their growth curve and to seek out a healthcare professional who could help you assess your child's health without stigma. Additionally, find an opportunity to talk about weight bias with your child and potentially implement lifestyle changes at home if you decide that they are needed and are the right step to support your child's health.

RULES ABOUT HOW MUCH TO EAT

In general, we want to avoid pressuring kids to eat. However, if you discover that your child is being influenced by friends or the media to restrict what they are eating, or if you see that they are experimenting with restricting how much they eat, you might want to consider creating some temporary rules around how much food they must eat, such as everyone needing to finish their plate at meals or everyone needing to be present for all meals whenever they are home.

This approach might be effective for children who:

- may be experimenting with restriction
- struggle with feeling or responding to fullness

This might be riskier for children who:

- have a good sense of interoception
- have anxiety-related appetite loss

Creating rules may be a good short-term approach to ensure that kids are not restricting, but mandating that a child must finish their plate isn't a long-term solution. As your child gets older, they will likely have fewer meals at home, and you won't be there to make sure they finish their food. So the root issues need to be addressed. Chapter 2 has ideas for minimizing exposure to the thin ideal and talking to kids about the thin ideal and media. If you believe that your child is being influenced by friends or peers to internalize the thin ideal, it can be helpful to talk to them about the idea that their friends may be getting harmful ideas from diet culture. A conversation might look like this:

⟦*Parent overhears their child's friend telling her today is a "cheat day," so she can take a break from her diet and have dessert with dinner and chips with lunch.*⟧

Parent: "I heard your friend mention 'cheat days.' You need to know that diets and 'cheat days' are not safe for kids. You and I together can decide when it makes sense to have chips and dessert."

Or

[*Parent overhears one child telling another child they didn't want a snack because they had to "save" calories for dinner.*]
Parent: "I heard your friend mention calories today."
Ten-year-old: "Yeah, Riley's on a diet, but her parents don't know."
Parent: "Tracking calories is part of diet culture. Diet culture is based on the idea that everyone should be thin, but people actually come in all shapes and sizes. Diet culture can make us very sick. Keeping track of calories makes it hard for kids to listen to what their bodies need and can be dangerous. It's not something that's safe for you to do. If you have questions about it or want to talk about diets, just let me know. You'll never get in trouble for talking about these things."

Or

[*Parent has been noticing their child has been eating less and less and has also made some comments that make them think their child might be concerned about gaining weight.*]
Twelve-year-old: "I can't finish my dinner."
Parent: "Why not?"
Twelve-year-old: "It will make me gain weight."
Parent: "Tell me more about that . . ."
. . .
Parent: "Thanks for explaining that to me. We're going to make sure we're healthy, which means we're going to make sure you eat enough to learn, grow, and play. You'll need to

finish your plate of food before leaving the table; we can play a game while you're finishing up."

Or

Fourteen-year-old: "Can we get some of these shakes?"
Parent: "Hmm. Where did you hear about these?"
Fourteen-year-old: "A bunch of my friends have them for lunch."
Parent: "Shakes can be good at times. It looks like these are for weight loss. Are your friends trying to lose weight?"
Fourteen-year-old: "A couple of them."
Parent: "Eating real, solid food for all your meals is important to make sure you get everything you need. We can keep some protein drinks in the house in case you want the option of having an emergency snack in your backpack, but diet shakes aren't for teens—that's the diet industry pushing kids to think they always need to be thinner and to buy their special drinks. We're not going to skip meals."

If you are going to set rules around how much a child must eat, don't serve any more than your child usually would have eaten. Additionally, if there is a certain food they dislike and generally won't eat, consider not serving that food during this period. This isn't a time to also try to treat picky eating.

Finally, be clear that your child is not in trouble—these rules are about helping them learn to listen to their body. Be warm and supportive and stay with them at the table (or wherever you're eating) while they are finishing their meal.

GET PROFESSIONAL HELP FOR DISORDERED EATING

If your child is showing signs of more serious disordered eating or an eating disorder, it's advisable to seek the help of a medical professional who can advise on a plan of action for your child. This could include their doctor, an eating disorder therapist, psychologist, or other professional with training in managing eating disorders. Signs for concern include noticing that your child is sneaking food, binge-ing, losing weight, restricting how much they are eating, skipping meals, tracking nutrients or calories, showing an unusual interest in nutrition, following new food "rules" (such as what foods they are allowed to eat and what foods they aren't), vomiting or laxa-tive use after meals (always going to the bathroom after meals / spending a lot of time in the bathroom), or excessive exercise to make up for food that was eaten. Often parents underestimate the severity of their child's symptoms or may feel guilt or shame around their child's eating struggles. Seeking help as soon as you suspect something will help reduce your child's risk of serious medical and psychological complications.

HIGH-RISK STRATEGIES TO AVOID

The following actions are very risky, and I do not recommend them.

ALLOWING YOUR CHILD TO PUT THEMSELF ON A DIET

It may be tempting to give in to a child if they say they want to go on a diet because their body is too big and their friends are making fun of them, but it's not safe for kids to put themselves on diets. If you have weight-related concerns, a better choice would be to seek help from a non-stigmatizing medical or eating disorder pro-fessional and talk to them first without your child present.

MINIMIZING OR IGNORING WHAT IS HAPPENING

If your child tells you that their friends are restricting and they are curious about it, or if you notice any of the signs of disordered eat-ing mentioned above, it is not the time to ignore what is going on. It's also not the time to think, *It's just a phase*, or, *All kids do this at some point*. Sometimes when we see our child having challenges with disordered eating, we want to deny that there is really a problem because disordered eating can be scary. We may want to ignore the problem because it feels embarrassing or like we failed at something. This is a time to get comfortable with being uncomfortable and to use courage to face the problem. The earlier you can put your energy into finding support for your child, the better for their long-term health. If it helps you to put a positive spin on things, keep in mind that it can be better to face these issues now as opposed to in early adulthood, because your child is young and you can help guide them and build the skills they will need throughout their lives.

APPLYING THE SIX-STEP FRAMEWORK FOR LAUREN

Step 1: Separate fact from fiction. Between the comment from Lauren's healthcare provider about her needing to lose weight and the teasing incident at school, her parents feel sick about the situation. They don't really have any stories that are driving them; they are already focused on the facts—namely, that Lauren needs support—stat.

Step 2: Pick the priority. Lauren's moms list their priorities: their daughter's physical, emotional, and social needs; their family's ability to address the situation based on their resources; their own energy, time, and mental health. All these factors seem important, and they're having a hard time deciding what their top priority is. So they decide to observe more closely for a bit to see what's happening. They start to pay more attention to what Lauren is eating, and they notice she is eating vegetables but then picking at the rest of the meal and spreading it around the plate to look like she's finished. They also notice the weight teasing at school wasn't a onetime incident; it continues to happen. Still, they decide her nutritional status was the first priority.

Step 3: Brainstorm—with a twist. Lauren's parents make a list of options for addressing Lauren's eating. They consider continuing to let her choose how much to eat, paying her to eat more, rewarding her, and taking away privileges if she refuses to eat her meals.

Step 4: Take a risk reduction approach. Lauren's moms are committed to building up her trust in her body—but they want to do this while still making sure she actually *is* following her body's hunger and fullness signals. They decide to set a boundary for a limited amount of time: Lauren needs to finish her entire meal before leaving the table. They also commit to reinforcing the idea, whenever possible, that kids and adults need to eat full meals to be healthy. They're hoping that this will reduce the drama at mealtime and make her more cooperative, since they will be requiring her to finish her meals.

Step 5: Think like a scientist and start an experiment. Lauren's parents talk to her frequently about how important it is to eat full meals, and they let Lauren know that she will need to eat all the foods on her plate before she gets down from the table, not just the vegetables. Lauren initially pushes back on this rule, but eventually, she gets into the routine, and the family starts eating regular meals together again. After some time, Lauren's moms decide that they no longer need to have the rule about her being required to finish her plate.

Step 6: Celebrate your wins, then continue to tweak your experiment. Lauren's parents give themselves a pat on the back for tackling the first part of the problem—their daughter's refusal to finish her meals—and then dive right back into problem-solving. Lauren is still being teased at school, so her parents contact the school and start looking for support resources related to bullying.

Next, they contact Lauren's healthcare provider to discuss Lauren's health and to get a referral for therapy options in their area, since the bullying is taking an emotional toll on her. They specifically ask the healthcare provider to put a note in her chart that says, "Do not discuss weight with child present. Parents willing to discuss health/lifestyle topics or have a separate call without child present to discuss weight." They also start to look for opportunities to help Lauren understand the thin ideal and weight bias, as well as how to care for her body without trying to change its size. They know she will continue to face stigma and that they will need to continue to advocate for her and provide her with supports as she grows up.

14

HEALTH DIAGNOSES AND THERAPEUTIC DIETS

As a parent, it can be incredibly scary to have a doctor diagnose your child with a specific medical condition or express concerns about your child's health. But keep in mind that if you are in this situation, it means that you have already done a lot right. You are paying attention to your child's health and seeking out the advice of experts to get the help they need. Whether your child has a chronic health condition, severe food allergies, or a weight-related diagnosis, I hope that the scenarios and practical strategies I present in this chapter will help make things more manageable for you. My goal is to help you lessen your anxiety and your child's anxiety, and, hopefully, to increase their cooperation if you need to alter what they eat. Diet changes—and talking to your child about them—can be overwhelming when you are just at the start of managing a health condition. Be kind to yourself and seek out support. It can make a world of difference.

Margot

Margot is an eight-year-old who has been in the ninetieth percentile for BMI most of her life. She eats a pretty standard diet, runs around outside at school, and tends to stay up late. She and her dad moved to a new city about a year ago, and since then, her dad has watched her eat larger amounts of cookies, chips, candy, and other hyperpalatable foods and rapidly gain weight. He's always taken a weight-neutral approach to bodies and body size at home, and the change in Margot's eating and weight are concerning. At her most recent checkup, her healthcare provider said, "Her BMI is in the ninety-ninth percentile, so she has obesity. I recommend immediately signing her up for a weight-loss program, and we'll do additional blood work. We can schedule a weight check for three months from now." Margot's dad left this appointment feeling conflicted about the fact that the conversation was sprung on him, and he regrets that he couldn't prepare his daughter for the doctor's speech. He's also frustrated that he didn't get the opportunity before the appointment to share his concerns about Margot's eating with the doctor, and he doesn't want to sign her up for a weight-loss program without careful consideration. That seems risky to him.

WHAT'S GOING ON?

There are many different diagnoses that might require changing or reconsidering a child's diet. These conditions and diagnoses could include:

- High cholesterol
- Diabetes
- High blood pressure
- Celiac disease
- Nonalcoholic fatty liver disease
- Overweight or obesity
- Allergies

- Asthma
- ADHD
- ASD
- Cystic fibrosis
- Cancer

In each of these cases, the causes—and the protocol to address the issue—will be very different. Still, there are some commonalities to keep in mind as you plan your path forward.

START WITH THE BASICS

If your child has a diagnosis or health concern, you already have a lot going on. And while it can be difficult for parents to nurture embodied independence in the best of circumstances, it's much harder if your child has, say, high cholesterol and needs to follow a diet to manage it. They may experience stigma or bias related to what they are eating and will need your support. Using the LoVE framework introduced in chapter 13, especially listening and validating, can help you support your child if they have negative peer experiences.

NUTRITION AND LIFESTYLE

Diet can be used to influence health conditions, and sometimes people use diet to treat specific conditions. A low-sodium diet, for example, has long been used to address hypertension, and a diet low in saturated fat and high in soluble fiber is often recommended for high cholesterol. Dietitians might also recommend more specific medical diets for children with kidney disease, cystic fibrosis, or other conditions. As we know, weight-loss diets are often prescribed for high weight.

Additionally, there are diets meant to address behavior or

attention deficits that sound "revolutionary"—proponents talk about how the diet can "cure" a child of their condition. They usually involve eliminating certain foods or addressing many elements in the Refining and Individualizing Health Impact Tiers. While these diets may be powerful solutions to managing symptoms for some children, families sometimes put the cart before the horse when it comes to changing their children's diets. Rather than focusing on the first four Health Impact Tiers, they may focus on tiers 5 and 6, because the elements in those tiers are getting the most media attention with the biggest health claims.

For example, many parents of kids with ADHD ask me specifically whether dyes might be affecting their child. This is a valid and important consideration (yes, dyes can have visible behavioral effects on some children with and without ADHD), and something I recommend parents consider in tier 5 if they are unsure if their child is affected. Yet they may not be giving that same attention and curiosity to food choices that we know have a big impact on kids with ADHD—like getting enough protein, fat—especially omega-3 fatty acids—fruits and veggies, fiber, sleep, and movement; reducing hyperpalatable foods with sugar and sodium; drinking water; and all the other elements in tiers 1 through 4. This can also apply to some families who have been told by medical providers that their child needs to lose weight. Rather than jumping straight to a weight-loss diet—an extreme strategy that carries serious risks—most families would be better off focusing first on the Health Impact Tiers.

HOW TO TALK ABOUT HEALTH DIAGNOSES AND FOOD

There are a lot of facts your child needs to know if they have a health condition that requires dietary changes. Kids deserve to understand what's going on in their bodies and how food will affect them. The goal is to arm them with knowledge and self-advocacy skills, without adding unnecessary anxiety or fear. This is tricky, especially if a condition can have severe health effects, and as a parent, it can be hard to know what to say.

Additionally, if possible, we don't want to suddenly deprive kids of the variety of foods they used to eat before their diagnosis to the point of triggering reactance (causing them to try extra hard to eat the foods that have been cut out). Ideally, we want to get them on board with the diet changes that could improve their health. This means talking about what they *can* have, instead of just what they can't have.

SCRIPTS FOR TALKING ABOUT HEALTH ISSUES WITH YOUR CHILD

Allergies

A friend of mine, author Ina K. Chung, shared the language she's used with her daughter about food allergies on her social media account @theasianallergymom. Here's how she talks to her child about understanding that she has allergies:

"We have an immune system that protects us from sicknesses, right? A food allergy is when something different has happened to the immune system and it thinks that foods that are usually safe are somehow dangerous. If a person is allergic to, say, dairy, ⟦and⟧ eats some cheese or butter, their allergen, then they could have some really uncomfortable symptoms like itching or diarrhea. But sometimes these symptoms can be a big emergency, and they might need help at a hospital right away."

I especially love her explanation of a more serious reaction—she is honest that it could be serious enough to require the hospital, without going into gory details about what might happen to the child in the very worst-case scenario. Notably, she told me that she decided to stop telling kids with food allergies that reactions could "lead to death" because allergists say that fatal anaphylaxis is exceedingly rare, especially when caretakers are educated, prepared and have access to treatment.

I think we can do well to adopt her mindset as we approach scripts that discuss various medical conditions with kids and how they might affect dietary choices. What follows are some additional child-friendly scripts for describing various health conditions to your kids.

Hypertension

"Our blood moves through our blood vessels. How hard it pushes through is called *blood pressure*. High blood pressure can hurt our heart, kidneys, and brain. If high blood pressure isn't taken care of, it can lead to medical emergencies. Salt in foods makes it hard to lower blood pressure, but fruits and vegetables help lower blood pressure. That's why we're changing the foods we have at home."

High cholesterol

"Our blood has a type of fat in it called *cholesterol*. If there is too much of it, it can stick to blood vessel walls. If this happens for a long time, it can block blood to the heart or brain when someone is an adult, and that would be an emergency. Fruits, veggies, seeds, and whole grains help reduce the cholesterol in our blood, and foods like hamburgers and cheese can make it go up. That's why we're going to be learning to make some new meals that we like, that reduce cholesterol."

Obesity or being overweight

It is important to note that in the current weight-focused health-care system, "obesity" and "overweight" have been given "diagnostic codes." These are insurance codes that say a person has a disease. There is some debate about whether high weight should be classified as a disease, especially when there is natural variation of body size. People can be healthy and unhealthy at various body sizes. However, diagnostic codes are based on BMI percentiles, which is an unreliable method for determining the amount of fat a person has in their body and what their health status is.

Many argue that making weight a diagnosis reduces weight stigma, because it acknowledges genetics and environmental factors, and removes some of the intense focus on personal responsibility (a person "has obesity"; they are not "obese"); others argue it increases weight stigma by saying an entire group of people is now diseased and should be medically treated for the disease, furthering weight-focused healthcare and weight stigma. I can see both sides of this argument, and you can choose the language that resonates with you. In any case, the medical system is using diagnostic codes, so if a child has a weight-related diagnosis that their provider told them about, like Margot does, they will need you to help them understand this in as non-stigmatizing a way as possible. Here is some helpful language that you might use:

"*Obesity* is a word that doctors use to describe fat tissue that stores energy. If there is a lot of energy stored, they may call that amount *obesity*, which is what your doctor said to you. For some people, the extra energy storage makes other parts of their bodies work extra hard and can lead to health problems in the future. That is why your doctor brought this up and mentioned a 'weight-loss diet.' But your doctor didn't find any signs that your body is working extra hard right now and didn't ask us many questions about how we live. We're not going to worry about a weight-loss diet. Instead of doing that, we're going to make sure your body is getting everything it needs to be healthy now and in the future. We're going to meet with a dietitian and talk about whether it would be helpful for our family to make some changes for our health, and if so, we'll do them together."

Prediabetes

"There is always glucose (a type of sugar) in your blood—people call it *blood sugar*. It shouldn't be too high or too low. If your body doesn't have the tools to use it, though, blood sugar gets high and starts damaging the body. That's called *diabetes*. Right now, your blood sugar is a little bit high, but not high enough to be diabetes. It's called *prediabetes*. Your body isn't being damaged by very high blood sugar, so this is an important time for us to help your body get the blood sugar back to normal. We're going to start trying some new foods and learning what else can help our bodies."

STRUCTURED PERMISSION

If your child is eating too much of certain foods, and these foods are negatively affecting their health, they might benefit from the practice of structured permission, which we initially discussed in chapter 2. You can step in and provide the structure or limits needed. Parents often ask me about how to handle situations where their child already has a higher weight, and then they begin gaining more rapidly because of eating large amounts of hyperpalatable foods. This situation can develop when a parent has allowed their child to choose how much to eat. These parents are typically not concerned about this from a body size perspective but from a health perspective. When a child begins eating more than their body needs, there may be an underlying reason, and rapid weight gain can contribute to other health problems.

Regardless of your child's weight, if they are gaining or losing weight unexpectedly, or if they have a medical condition that requires dietary restrictions, structured permission may be the way to help them get in touch with their body. This could look like taking a break from purchasing some foods, changing what foods are routinely available at home, limiting how much your child is allowed to eat of certain foods, or having a firmer eating routine.

PROBLEM-SOLVING STRATEGIES TO TRY

USING SUPPLEMENTS TO TREAT NUTRIENT DEFICIENCIES

This may be effective for children who:

- have a known deficiency
- have poor weight gain
- have access to supplements

This may be riskier for children who:

- don't have a health practitioner overseeing their care, especially if the child has more serious health conditions

If your child is chronically not getting enough of a nutrient, they may have an insufficiency (low levels but not causing major health issues or disease) or a deficiency (very low levels that are causing major health issues or disease). These can only be detected through clinical testing. Two children can consume the same diet, but due to differences in how our bodies absorb, use, and store certain nutrients, one child may develop a deficiency and the other may not. Spotting a nutrient deficiency can be tricky. Common symptoms include weight loss, growth changes, appetite loss, fatigue, low energy, sluggishness, weakness, slow wound healing, itchy dry skin, pale skin, and brittle nails.

If you suspect that your child has a deficiency, ask your healthcare provider about ordering blood work to test your child's nutrient levels. This way, you will have the facts, and you can avoid under- or over-supplementing, which can occur when you make the supplementation decision entirely on your own. If you want to gather additional information about your child's diet before making this request for blood work, or if your child's healthcare provider is hesitant to do blood work, you can track what your child eats for three to seven days to find out what nutrients they are getting and compare that with the recommended intakes.

If you discover a large gap between the recommended intake of a nutrient and what your child is eating, it can be a clue that they aren't getting what they need and may be more likely to have a deficiency. If blood work shows that your child has an insufficiency or deficiency, they will likely need a supplement to have their nutrient levels restored. They may also need a regular maintenance dose of the supplement to prevent them from becoming deficient again. Bear in mind that children's multivitamins do not usually contain doses of nutrients that will resolve a deficiency, and the doses that it takes to overcome a deficiency are sometimes not safe to take long term.

If you decide to introduce supplements, make sure to use third-party tested supplements as discussed in chapter 5. If your supplements come in the form of a nutritional drink, try serving it after dinner. Otherwise, your child may fill up on the drink and not eat their meals. Finally, I highly recommend working with a healthcare provider if your child has a deficiency. Replenishing nutrients to resolve a deficiency can come with risks, and even I check in with my kids' doctors or consult with a licensed pediatric nutritionist or dietitian (one that specifically has experience with nutrient repletion) if I'm trying to resolve a deficiency with one of my kids.

USING SUPPLEMENTS TO MANAGE HEALTH CONDITIONS

This may be effective for children who:

- have a condition that is known to respond to supplements
- have a provider experienced in treating the condition with supplements
- have access to supplements

This may be riskier for children who:

- have no practitioner overseeing their care, especially if the child has more serious health conditions

Supplements are part of some children's regular healthcare protocol. When we talk about managing health conditions, supplements can be used in a way that is similar to the way medications might be used to address a specific health issue. It's important to think about therapeutic supplementation in this way, because a common belief is that if a supplement is "natural," it can't have negative side effects. This is not true. When vitamins, minerals, or other supplements that alter body chemistry are not used properly, there can be dangerous side effects. It is important to think critically about the way we decide to use medications and supplements and allow our children to use them. The pharmaceutical and supplement industries are both extremely lucrative, with histories of marketing and manipulating the way scientific research is reported for profit—often at the expense of our health. So be wary of their claims, and be a smart consumer.

My belief is that each family can decide whether to use supplements and/or medications based on their preferences and their child's needs. The key is understanding that nutritional supplements can have risks, just like medications. If you decide to use supplements for managing your child's health condition, it's important to work with a specialist who has experience treating this condition in children—just as you would if you were using medications. I highly recommend choosing a specialist who is accountable to a credentialing body or who has a license to practice. This usually means they must follow an ethics policy (important!) and that they complete continuing education relevant to their practice.

This is not, in my view, the time to work with someone who has a five-week online certificate, to follow the advice laid out in a blog article by a wellness influencer, or even to take the advice of a doctor who hasn't practiced medicine in the last ten years because they became an influencer and started selling supplements. It's also not the time to rely on a credentialed person who doesn't have specific training and experience in the condition your child has. For example, I am a registered dietitian. There is an organization that certifies my credential and requires ethics agreements, and they make sure I do my continuing education requirements to keep my credential. But I don't have training or experience in how to use supplements to help children manage conditions. I could *tell* you I am qualified because I'm a registered dietitian nutritionist, but I don't believe I am, because this is not my area of expertise.

It would be better either to find a registered dietitian nutritionist (RDN) who has specialized in integrative and functional medicine and has experience working with children or to work with a certified nutrition specialist (CNS) with experience working with children. These practitioners specialize in using food and supplements to support health and treat health conditions. Both require extensive training and experience, have continuing education requirements, and are accountable to a credentialing body and licensing requirements in most states.

I once attended a continuing education class where the speaker explained that the mark of a responsible professional treating with supplements is that they will tell you when you can stop taking them or suggest specific tests to see if you still need to take them (for example, routinely testing vitamin D levels). If someone is recommending that you put your child on a lot of supplements without any ongoing testing, clear rationale, or "end date" to those supplements, especially if they're financially benefiting from the sale of those supplements, it's a good time to be skeptical of the treatment and the practitioner. You might consider getting a second opinion.

USING THERAPEUTIC DIETS TO MANAGE HEALTH CONDITIONS

This may be effective for children who:

- are willing to eat enough foods in a therapeutic diet to meet their nutrient needs
- have practitioner observation
- have ADHD, hypertension, high cholesterol, type 2 diabetes, nonalcoholic fatty liver disease, ASD, or other conditions for which some children have responded to a therapeutic diet

This may be riskier for children who:

- have disordered eating
- are extremely picky

What we eat can be very powerful, and when certain things are added or taken out, a child's health can be altered. At the same time, when therapeutic diets—defined as eating or excluding foods for the purpose of addressing a specific health concern—become popular, some of the details are often not adequately communicated, such as the specific group of people who may benefit from the diet or how the diet should be conducted. For example, it's currently somewhat common to hear a "gluten-free, dairy-free" diet recommended to manage health conditions, including eczema, autism, or others, in children. Proponents of this diet will offer stories of the many kids who have benefited from it, the biological reasons for why it works, and even some research studies to back it up. However, it is important to keep in mind that when we remove entire categories of foods from children's diets, it can negatively impact their health; it reduces variety, which can cause nutrient deficiencies or new health problems; and it also has the potential for complicating embodiment or a child's relationship with food. Additionally, the diets don't work for many of the children who are put on them.

If you have decided to put your child on a therapeutic diet, to the extent possible, I would recommend working with a healthcare professional before starting to help monitor your child's health status. If you are going to remove a food or follow an elimination diet, make sure there are enough substitutions that your child will be able to meet all their nutrient needs. This means that you can financially afford the substitutions, your child will actually eat them, and you have the time and energy to make sure they have them. If your child will not eat any of the substitutions, then it may be dangerous to eliminate foods from their diet.

If you decide to go ahead with the substitution, speak factually to your child about the changes you're making. This will help them understand why it's happening and what they can expect, even if they aren't excited about the change. Avoid language like, "This is bad for you," "Those foods are unhealthy," or "These foods will make you better ⟦or make your condition go away⟧," as these may lay the groundwork for broken promises or guilt if the diet doesn't work. Instead, take this as an opportunity to help your child embrace the message: "I can listen to my body to find out how to eat best for me." You might say something like, "We're going to see how we feel when we eat these new foods," or "You've been having those tummy aches—it might be because your body needs more of some foods, so we're going to be eating more XYZ for the next few weeks to find out how it feels."

The "we" in those quotes is important. Rather than removing a food from just your child's diet, consider whether the rest of the family could also make the change as a form of support. If your child has allergies or a condition like cystic fibrosis, they may need a specialized diet that is not practical for the whole family. If, on the other hand, your child needs to adjust their diet to manage high cholesterol, that can be a family affair.

If you do decide to remove foods, it's important to use Step 5: Think Like a Scientist and Start an Experiment from our six-step feeding dilemma framework—this will help you determine whether the diet is actually working. Write down what you observe after your child starts the diet. Ideally, you and any other adults in the home would write down their observations separately, and someone from outside the home who observes the child would also write down their observations. Do the experimental diet for a set period (like two to four weeks, unless a longer trial period is suggested by a healthcare practitioner), go back to a "normal" diet for a set period of time (two to four weeks), and observe what happens. Then do the experimental diet *again* to see if what you observed the first time still happens the second time.

For example, perhaps a parent decided they wanted to try a gluten- and dairy-free diet to address their child's eczema. They would perhaps take pictures of the eczema patches, then do the diet for a set period of time, then take more pictures, compare the two, and do it all again, starting with a regular diet. Then, based on their observations, they would decide how to move forward.

It's easy to be biased and see changes that aren't there. In the case of the example above, the parent might compare the pictures and then ask a friend to compare them as well, and only then would they decide whether the diet made a change. Repeating the experiment twice and having as many people as possible share observations can help decrease that bias and keep you from having to unnecessarily restrict your child from foods.

Once the change has been implemented, it's important to also pay attention to how your child is responding emotionally to the new diet. It can be upsetting to have all your foods suddenly change! It might also cause reactions in some children. Use a listening strategy (such as the LoVE framework in chapter 13) to have tricky conversations.

HOLDING FIRM BOUNDARIES IF YOUR CHILD'S HEALTH IS AT RISK

This may be effective for children who:*

- have a medical condition
- are not significantly meeting their nutrient needs
- are having health problems because of their eating
- have executive function difficulties such as poor impulse control

This may be riskier for children with:

- increased risk of eating disorders
- feelings of shame or guilt about food, their bodies, or their appetites
- past food insecurity

---

* Firm boundaries may be recommended as part of eating disorder therapy and genetic appetite disorders. Treatment of those disorders is best handled with a team of healthcare professionals who can advise on the best interventions for your child. They will not be discussed in this section.

Sometimes there are particular foods or amounts of foods that kids cannot have for health reasons. In this case, firm boundaries—like not purchasing a certain food or keeping it locked in a cabinet—may be needed. (For a reminder of how to mitigate the serious risks of firm boundaries, see chapter 11.)

CHANGING YOUR CHILD'S DIET FOR WEIGHT LOSS OR WEIGHT MAINTENANCE

This may be effective for children who:

- are at high risk for or who already have health conditions that may be influenced by their weight
- who are unexpectedly and significantly increasing in BMI percentiles for an extended period*

This may be riskier for children who:

- have eating disorders or disordered eating
- have a family history of disordered eating

Margot's dad had some concerns about putting his daughter on a weight-loss plan, as many parents probably would. The truth is, there isn't much research on whether weight-loss programs contribute to eating disorders. Many eating disorder therapists advise against weight-loss programs for children for this reason, although there is some research to suggest that if a child participates in a structured and professionally run weight-loss program, it can decrease the risk of developing an eating disorder. If you do decide

---

* While BMI alone is a poor measure of health, BMI *percentiles* can help identify unexpected increases or decreases in a child's growth trajectories that may be a symptom of underlying changes to behavior or health.

to take this approach to reduce the risk for disordered eating, it's important to work with a qualified professional (an eating disorder therapist, a dietitian, or a physician), focus on health over weight loss, and do as much as you can to nurture your child's embodied independence.

If you decide to implement a weight-loss diet, your child should still be able to eat until they are full. Be wary of allowing them to use a tracking app to monitor their food intake or weight loss. Pay attention to whether they may be posting body shape selfies on social media, using image altering apps or AI, or following weight-loss focused "thinspiration," "pro-ana" (pro anorexia nervosa), "pro-mia" (pro bulimia nervosa), or "skinnytok" content on social media. This kind of content is harmful, increasing your child's internalized weight bias, encouraging them to use disordered eating strategies, and potentially boosting their shame and anxiety related to their body. Additionally, make sure the weight-loss diet your child is on embraces all foods, including foods purely for enjoyment. Remember, being able to enjoy all foods is a core component of a healthy relationship with food. You should also make sure your child has clothes that fit properly, without being constricting or suggesting that they need to change their body to fit their clothes.

Children like Margot who are put on weight-loss diets by healthcare professionals will likely have other symptoms like hypertension, prediabetes, movement impairment, or metabolic syndrome. If this is the case, your child does not need to hear, "You need to lose fifteen pounds to lower your BMI." They need to hear factual information about their body from their healthcare providers or parents like, "Right now your kidneys are working extra hard, and eating certain foods can help them relax," or "Your body needs to have more of some nutrients to work best." If you are implementing a specific diet to support a health condition, take this opportunity to discuss what different foods do in the body. For example, certain eating patterns like the DASH (Dietary Approaches to Stop Hypertension) diet have been shown to lower high blood pressure. Learning about which nutrients support blood pressure, such as potassium and magnesium, and which foods have those nutrients, may help reframe eating changes away from "calories" to "foods that do stuff in my body."

Remember, you don't have to focus your child's entire life on weight to make changes to improve everyone's health. You don't have to discuss body size or shape. You don't have to have a scale out all the time (even if weighing is sometimes required, you could use a scale without a screen that syncs weight to an app rather than displaying it). You don't have to discuss weight loss at the family meal. If your child wants to discuss it, of course you can, but it doesn't need to be a frequent topic of conversation. And as always, if you are implementing any sort of restrictive food plan, watch for disordered eating or thinking. If your child starts to exhibit signs of disordered eating, seek out the help of an eating disorder therapist right away to support them further.

TREATMENT THAT INCLUDES GLP-1 INHIBITORS

GLP-1 inhibitors are medications used for weight loss. At this time, some of the medications have been approved for children ages twelve and up, with newer clinical trial data that may be used to expand their use to six-to-eleven-year-olds. There is only a small amount of research at this time on using these medications with children, or on the rates of disordered eating by children who use them. But the evidence base is growing. Barring dangerous side effects or new information about risks of long-term use, we can safely assume that these drugs will become commonplace.

I attended a medical conference a few years ago and went to a session about treatments for childhood obesity. One pediatrician (who disclosed that she is often sponsored to speak by the pharmaceutical companies making GLP-1 medications, although not at that session) said very clearly, "My goal is to help every pediatrician start prescribing weight-loss medications." The spread of GLP-1 use among children is inevitable, regardless of whether you are for or against it. Plus, children are already exposed to mass marketing campaigns for weight-loss medications on TV, mail, music streaming apps, and in other media. So, in addition to approaching weight loss with a focus on embodied independence, we also need a way to explain the purpose of these medications to children. I like the way my friend explained it to her daughter when she asked about a billboard advertising GLP-1 inhibitors: "Fat is stored energy. Sometimes people decide with their doctors that some of that energy needs to be let go, and medications help that happen."

HIGH-RISK STRATEGIES TO AVOID

The following actions are very risky, and I don't recommend them, as it is difficult or impossible to reduce the risks.

TALKING ABOUT BODY SHAPE/SIZE TO GET YOUR CHILD TO EAT DIFFERENTLY

This may seem like a strange thing to advise against in a chapter that addresses choosing to pursue weight loss for your child. I can't ignore the research, however, which indicates that discussing a child's body shape puts them at greater risk for developing an eating disorder. It is unknown if discussing body size or shape in the context of medical care is different from casually discussing your child's body at the dinner table.

LETTING YOUR CHILD START AND PLAN THEIR OWN WEIGHT-LOSS DIET

Researchers have observed that kids who put themselves on a diet are more likely to have disordered eating, depressive symptoms, overeating, and greater weight gain over time. If you have decided to pursue weight loss for your child and are not involving a professional, at the very least be actively involved so that you can help prevent them from participating in unhealthy or extreme weight control strategies.

PUNISHING YOUR CHILD FOR REFUSING CERTAIN FOODS

For kids with diagnoses, making diet changes may not be fun. They may resist these changes, and adding punishment when they won't eat certain foods is not going to make eating an enjoyable experience that builds connection for the family.

LETTING A CHILD BE HUNGRY FOR THE SAKE OF WEIGHT LOSS

Children should never be excessively hungry during treatment for weight loss or maintenance, beyond the mild hunger that all kids benefit from before meals or snacks. Hunger triggers negative responses from the body, which will not only increase a child's risk of gaining weight in the future but can also be psychologically damaging.

APPLYING THE SIX-STEP FRAMEWORK FOR MARGOT

Step 1: Separate fact from fiction. Margot's dad is caught off guard by her pediatrician's comments and initially feels discouraged by them. He begins to doubt his parenting skills, believing that this is just proof that he's not a good parent. But then he takes a beat and decides to focus on the facts. His daughter needs some specific care, and he needs to learn what he can do to support her.

Step 2: Pick the priority. There is a lot going on in this family's life. Margot's dad considers all the elements of his daughter's health and lists them as priorities: her weight, her future risk of disease, his capacity as a parent, and her internalized weight bias—especially after their disturbing meeting with the doctor. He decides that the number one priority is to address her health.

Step 3: Brainstorm—with a twist. Margot's dad considers and lists the different potential ways of communicating with Margot about the issue, and he plans to contact a registered dietitian for support.

Step 4: Take a risk reduction approach. Margot's dad continues to be concerned about her embodiment and decides to prioritize avoiding any unnecessary discussion about weight or size. This includes finding a dietitian who is on board with health-focused instead of weight-focused treatment, contacting the doctor's office, and making decisions based on Margot's mental and physical health needs, not weight-loss goals. It also includes talking to Margot about the healthcare appointment to try to get her on board.

Step 5: Think like a scientist and start an experiment. Margot's dad has a conversation with his daughter about the doctor's comments. He helps her understand what *obesity* means in the medical context. He also listens to his daughter's take on the doctor's appointment and validates her concerns. Since he doesn't have all the necessary knowledge to assess Margot's diet, he contacts his health insurance company and finds out that dietitian services are covered if a person has been diagnosed with obesity.

Margot's dad finds a pediatric dietitian in the area and communicates his desire to avoid discussing or focusing on Margot's body weight or size. He also explains that he wants to learn more about whether they should take a more therapeutic approach to her diet. The dietitian does an initial nutrition assessment with Margot (without weighing her) and determines that she is not eating the recommended amounts of fruits, vegetables, and whole grains, and is consuming too many added sugars and too much sodium. When the dietitian discusses the assessment results, she does so without Margot present, so she can openly discuss potential contributors to weight gain. The dietitian also notes that the timing of Margot's change in eating came right after a stressful life event—moving. Margot's dad considers his own tendency to stress-eat, and suddenly Margot's eating makes sense.

Margot's blood work comes back: Her cholesterol is borderline high, she is deficient in vitamin D, and she is low on iron. Margot's dad works with her doctor and dietitian to use supplements to restore her vitamin D and iron. Based on her borderline high cholesterol, Margot's dad decides to implement a therapeutic diet at home and to eliminate hyperpalatable foods. He explains to Margot what *high cholesterol* means and tells her they will be eating differently to try to address it. He removes all hyperpalatable food from the house to make it easier to eat the foods they need to eat. He keeps an eye out for how Margot is handling the changes.

Step 6: Celebrate your wins, then continue to tweak your experiment. Margot's dad is happy with the information he's gained and the progress that they are making, and he takes a minute to feel a sense of accomplishment. He continues tweaking his experiment, however. Margot learns to eat the new recipes and high-fiber foods, and she finds that she enjoys them. She remains obsessed with cookies, chips, and candy, however, constantly asking for these foods. When she gets them elsewhere, she will eat as much as she can and sneak some back home. Margot's dad isn't comfortable with this and suspects the restrictive diet is triggering ongoing reactance. He's also not confident he can hold the boundaries long term, which would be necessary to end the reactance.

Margot's dad discusses the issue with her and explains that she doesn't need to sneak eating around him. He understands that she would still like to be able to have fun foods at home and notes that they still need to find a way to support her body with other foods. He is careful to avoid any qualifications involving her weight and body during this conversation. Margot and her dad decide they will have dessert every night and chips with lunches. While this is more hyperpalatable food than Margot's dad would like, he gets her buy-in, and this is a good strategy for them for now. He plans to reduce how often he serves chips and dessert in the future, and he thinks a slower approach to change is a better fit for his family.

Finally, Margot's dad starts learning new strategies—instead of eating—for handling his own anxiety. He starts to model these strategies and teaches Margot how to use them as well, which becomes a bonding activity for them in addition to helping them both manage their stress. Margot's weight and cholesterol continue to be monitored by her healthcare provider, but her dad does not allow the provider to discuss her weight during appointments. They focus on how she feels and the actions she is taking to improve her health.

CONCLUSION

The Courage to Feed ***Your*** Child

Whenever I give a podcast interview, it almost always ends with the interviewer asking me if there's "anything else" I'd like to share with parents. And the answer is always, yes, there is.

Here's what I want to leave you with: I know you're capable. The fire hose of information giving you all the "right" answers can easily drown out your confidence and certainty—it's constantly telling you that you don't know enough, that you aren't doing enough, and that whatever you're doing, you're doing it wrong. But the truth is, you're doing lots of things right, even if you are exploring alternative solutions to problems or want to make some changes.

You don't have to be certain to be courageous. We are all desperate for certainty, especially when it comes to raising our kids in the best way possible. In a complicated and rapidly changing world like ours, however, where profits are prioritized over the health of our families and extreme health recommendations get the most media attention, strategies that we can be certain about are in short supply. So much of the health- and diet-related information we are exposed to is designed to make us crave the very certainty that we can't have when it comes to feeding our kids—and then to offer us someone else's certainty at a price.

Certainty can be dangerous. It can lead us to narrow-minded thinking and solutions, or no solutions at all. Certainty feeds the belief that if we know the right answer, everyone else must be wrong. It's all too easy to say, "I'll never be able to do it right," when there's only a "right" and "wrong" way to feed kids. Courage, on the other hand, gives us space. It allows us to believe that a way forward is out there, and it pushes us to go find that way forward even when it's scary or uncomfortable. When we have courage, we can consider our child and our family, and we can give ourselves the space to be curious. We can ask, "What if I *can* get them what they need?" "What if I try this?" and "What matters most to *us* here?" When we ask these courageous questions, we move toward solutions. As it turns out, we should welcome uncertainty, because uncertainty is an invitation to courage—the courage we need in the unpredictable adventure of feeding our kids.

In this moment, as you consider which of the tools in this book might be right for your family, I hope that you *aren't* feeling the warm fuzzies of a "you got this" pep talk. Instead, I hope you feel the burn of the ever-growing courage inside of you. This is the courage that will enable you to put in the effort to feed your child, and to find joy and connection eating with them. It's the courage that will allow you to embrace a positive mindset about feeding your child. It's the courage you'll need to support your child when situations arise that you would never have chosen or asked for. This courage will help you to embrace nuance and make complicated decisions—and to change what you're doing when it's not working for your family without feeling guilty. This is the courage that will enable you to acknowledge the truth if feeding your child isn't going so well, to look for the resources you need, and to find creative ways to steer things back in a better direction. This courage will allow you to embrace and celebrate each of your family's successes as gifts that your child will take with them into adulthood.

ACKNOWLEDGMENTS

I am deeply grateful for the opportunity to write this book and to the many people who made it possible.

First, I'm grateful for the Kids Eat in Color social media community. I started Kids Eat in Color in a moment where I wondered if I was alone, and it has been the gift of a lifetime to learn I'm not. None of this would have happened without each parent who worked hard at feeding their own child, used my resources, and also shared Kids Eat in Color with their friends, family, and communities.

I'm thankful to Macmillan and Flatiron for the amazing opportunity to create this book. Julie Will saw what parents needed in this book and didn't stop until we got it right. Sophie Garcia-Cubas Assemat walked with and advocated for me during a difficult time in my life: citation formatting. Her can-do energy is contagious. The team at Flatiron made every element of this book real: Emily Walters, Jeremy Pink, Kate Keating, Jonathan Sung, Roxanne Jones, Laywan Kwan, and Leah Carlson-Stanisic. An extra shout-out to the parents at Flatiron who live the daily juggle of making meaningful books a reality and feeding their own kids.

I'm grateful to those who brought out the best in this book. David Doerrer saw the possibility of a book, opened the door, and tolerated my two emails to every one of his. Rachel Bertsche's insights and editing made this book even more powerful, and she brought order to tens of thousands of words of chaos at the start. Jessica Snider looked at the big picture at a key moment and drew out the strengths in the narrative.

Paul Anderson is my favorite (and only) husband. We got to celebrate our twentieth wedding anniversary with a work date to keep ahead of our respective book- and exam-writing deadlines, and it was perfect. It's trite to say this book wouldn't have been possible without him—he played a crucial role. I wouldn't have read the research with the critical eye that makes this book what it is and there would be no practice of curiosity. He held down the fort while I wrote and always tells me he will never bet against me, even in the ups and downs. He lost sleep working at night so that he could do school pickup and drop-off and countless other kid-related tasks and I could write for extra hours. He took the brunt of how much I "verbally processed" (talked incessantly about) every topic I wrote about. He asked me crucial questions about the details, which showed me what I needed to fix for readers' benefit. He's a great pal.

It is one of my greatest privileges to be the mom of my kids and learn to feed them, and I am grateful to them for their support. M.S.'s creative spark brings endless energy, art, and laughter to my world. M.B. inspires me to never give up on seemingly impossible ambitions until they are a reality.

I'm grateful for the Kids Eat in Color team, who passionately supports families and their children's health with skill, empathy, and care. They are the most positive, above and beyond people you will find and I'm lucky to work with them. Molly, Carrie, Jenn, and Olivia make sure parents feel heard and taken care of. Sasha Martinez Larkin and Tiffany Cipullo read so many iterations of this book over the past two years. They provided feedback, made sure the text sounded as friendly and nonjudgmental as I meant it, and cheered me on at every step. They handled everything else when I needed to write, jumped in on the weekends, and turned my abstract ideas into real-life tangible supports for families. Their insight, positivity, and hard work have made Kids Eat in Color what it is. C. J. Stermer wholeheartedly dove in, energized the team, created a seamless experience for families, and made sure all the bows got tied.

The deep research base for this book, pulled together in a short time, was only possible with a team. Researchers Dr. Coline Couillault, Dr. Aubrey Moore, Dr. Elizabeth Denbow, Dr. Johanna Hanley, and Jennifer Kasyan, MEd, helped me sort through thousands of citations and deeply analyze research literature so that this book could have the strongest foundation possible.

I have the pleasure of working with an incredibly skilled and intelligent group of specialists. Nooshin Kiankhooy, CEDS-C, LCPC, and Amanda Bechtel, ATR-BC, LCPC, LCPAT, shared their insight and experiences as eating disorders therapists and parents, and provided feedback on book sections about disordered eating and body image. Hyemyung Kim, RD, CDN, CNSC, CLC, contributed her specialized knowledge in infant feeding to the chapter on starting the feeding journey. Dr. Christine Lippard helped me understand child education and inspires me with her practice of curiosity in the face of feeding dilemmas. Dr. Alexandria Delozier taught me that information gives children autonomy and autonomy bolsters mental health. Dr. Katie Kaenkumchorn provided gastroenterology expertise. Laura Petix, MS, OTR/L, and Erinn Jacobi, MS, OTR/L, shared their expertise on the child sensory system and emotional regulation. Stefanie Kain, MEd, shared her insight on child development, learning, and education. My anonymous scientist friend shared her expertise on water and health, inspires me daily with her intentional lifestyle, and her kids kept my kids busy for hundreds of afternoons.

The support of friends has helped me be the person I've needed to be to write this book, and I'm grateful to them. Ann, Allison, Maria, Marielle, Ron, Annie, Sara, and Katherine teach me to see the possibilities and magic in life. Melissa, Gene, Krista, Gar, Ashton, and Jim held space for me during a crucial time. Lori Martin helped me (and our entire family) stay sane with logistical support and consistent presence. Agata Williams helps me stay my own person, now and in early motherhood. Susie Allison warned me and provided encouragement, feedback, and generous support for the book anyway. Ashley Nowe helped me build muscle and stay regulated. Caitlin Self helped me get over an iron deficiency expeditiously so I could think clearly again.

There are also people who provided key guidance at turning points in my life that undergird what is written here. Dr. Yaffe set the tone for Kids Eat in Color and this book by teaching me not to "should" on myself. Dr. Griffin told me to study people. Dr. Arnold told me to go to graduate school. Dr. Peterson told me not to follow a traditional nutrition path. Dr. Gittelsohn gave me an independent study when I needed one, which taught me how to do a mean literature review. Dr. Freeman made the writing of this book possible. Marisol Colette helped me own my role and appreciate silk.

Tens of thousands of family meals with incredible people from five generations have shaped me and shown me what family meals are capable of. I am grateful to those who have been at those meals. My siblings Evan, Emily, Ryan, and David, helped me master division at a young age so that we all got the same number of cookies. They, along with my extended siblings Rachel, Gene, Caro, and Melissa, and nieces and nephew, have given my kids the richest and most exciting family meal experiences, just like I've had rich and exciting meal experiences with my aunts, uncles, and cousins (the infamous cousin "junk food" party deserves an honorable mention). My dad taught me to "Go big or go home" and love futomaki. My mom fed me for eighteen years, filled the freezer with soups to keep everyone fed while I was writing, and never ever forgets that I don't like mayo. My in-laws Tim and Eunice have been supportive of all our holiday hosting over the years, whether bare minimum or extra fancy. They give my kids the experience of holiday cookie decorating and family food history that I never could. They watched the kids many nights so Paul and I could connect amid the chaos of the past few years. My grandma Perl understood that ice cream and business supplies solve every problem. My grandpa Perl's garden embedded a deep love of macadamia nuts, green beans, figs, and beets. My granddad Adams taught us that oatmeal served properly is an art, science, and essential. My grandma Adams never pressured or guilted us for not eating her butter/margarine, peanut butter, and jelly sandwiches. My grandma-in-law Erna won my heart over lunch at a diner while we chatted about the one person we most loved to talk about—her favorite grandson and my out-of-town, soon-to-be fiancé. My great-grandma Scott sent magical date pinwheels from afar every Christmas. My great-grandma Fay passed down the family stubborn streak (that I put to use while writing this book) and won my love through hyperpalatable snacks and TV every Wednesday.

APPENDIX

Nutritional Needs

FIBER

Fiber recommendations vary for children because research on fiber and children is still developing. Some recommendations are easy to remember and calculate at the minimum level, and others are focused on optimal levels based on calories consumed and long-term health benefits.

MINIMUM RECOMMENDATION (AGE + 5 RULE)

For children ages 2 and older, a simple minimum is the child's age in years plus 5 grams per day:

Age 2: 7 g/day
Age 3: 8 g/day
Age 4: 9 g/day
Age 5: 10 g/day
Age 6: 11 g/day
Age 7: 12 g/day
Age 8: 13 g/day

For older children, continue adding 5 to their age, up to the following IOM Adequate Intake values.

OPTIMAL RECOMMENDATION (IOM ADEQUATE INTAKES)

1–3 years: 19 g/day
4–8 years: 25 g/day
9–13 years (males): 31 g/day
9–13 years (females): 26 g/day
14–18 years (males): 38 g/day
14–18 years (females): 26 g/day

CALCIUM

Calcium recommendations for children vary widely across different health authorities worldwide. These differences reflect various methodological approaches researchers use to study calcium needs, as well as potentially other influences such as regional dietary patterns and industry considerations. Below is a summary of recommendations from major health organizations, followed by a synthesis of the ranges by age group. The following reflect differences of opinion among different professional groups and health authorities.

SUMMARY OF RANGES BY AGE GROUP

1–3 years: 350–700 mg/day
4–6 years: 450–1000 mg/day
7–10 years: 550–1300 mg/day
11–14 years (males): 1000–1300 mg/day
11–14 years (females): 800–1300 mg/day

Here are specific recommendations by organization:

UNITED KINGDOM (UK DEPARTMENT OF HEALTH / SACN)

Reference Nutrient Intakes

1–3 years: 350 mg/day
4–6 years: 450 mg/day
7–10 years: 550 mg/day
11–18 years (females): 800 mg/day
11–18 years (males): 1000 mg/day

UNITED STATES AND CANADA (INSTITUTE OF MEDICINE)

Recommended Dietary Allowances

1–3 years: 700 mg/day
4–8 years: 1000 mg/day
9–18 years: 1300 mg/day

WORLD HEALTH ORGANIZATION (WHO/FAO)

Recommended Nutrient Intakes

1–3 years: 500 mg/day
4–6 years: 600 mg/day
7–9 years: 700 mg/day
10–18 years: 1300 mg/day

EUROPE (EUROPEAN FOOD SAFETY AUTHORITY)

Population Reference Intakes

1–3 years: 450 mg/day
4–10 years: 800 mg/day
11–17 years: 1150 mg/day

IRON

Iron recommendations are relatively similar around the world, and the Institute of Medicine recommendations are provided here.

RECOMMENDED DIETARY ALLOWANCES

7–12 months: 11 mg/day
1–3 years: 7 mg/day
4–8 years: 10 mg/day
9–13 years: 8 mg/day
14–18 years (males): 11 mg/day
14–18 years (females): 15 mg/day

NOTES

Introduction

4 ***billions of dollars:*** Jensen, M. L., McCann, M., Leming-Milici, F., Mancini, S., and Harris, J. L. (2022). FACTS 2022. Food industry self-regulation: Changes in nutrition of foods and drinks that may be advertised to children. *UConn Rudd Center for Food Policy & Health*; Federal Trade Commission. (2012). *Marketing Food to Children and Adolescents: A Review of Food Marketing to Children and Adolescents Follow-Up Report.*

4 **The more kids are exposed:** Ares, G., Antúnez, L., Alcaire, F., et al. (2025). Associations between exposure to digital food marketing and food consumption in adolescence: A cross-sectional study in an emerging country. *BMC Public Health, 25*(1). https://doi.org/10.1186/S12889-025-24443-Z; Arrona-Cardoza, P., Labonté, K., Cisneros-Franco, J. M., and Nielsen, D. E. (2023). The effects of food advertisements on food intake and neural activity: A systematic review and meta-analysis of recent experimental studies. *Advances in Nutrition, 14*(2), 339–351. https://doi.org/10.1016/j.advnut.2022.12.003; Bagnato, M., Roy-Gagnon, M. H., Vanderlee, L., White, C., Hammond, D., and Potvin Kent, M. (2023). The impact of fast food marketing on brand preferences and fast food intake of youth aged 10–17 across six countries. *BMC Public Health, 23*(1), 1436. https://doi.org/10.1186/s12889-023-16158-w.

4 **we see it on TV:** Bruce, A. S., Pruitt, S. W., Ha, O. R., et al. (2016). The influence of televised food commercials on children's food choices: Evidence from ventromedial prefrontal cortex activations. *Journal of Pediatrics, 177*, 27–32.e1. https://doi.org/10.1016/j.jpeds.2016.06.067; Nestle, M. (2013). *Food Politics: How the Food Industry Influences Nutrition and Health (10th ed.).* University of California Press; World Health Organization. (2023). *Policies to Protect Children from the Harmful Impact of Food Marketing WHO Guideline.*

4 **Tony the Tiger:** Mulligan, C., Remedios, L., Ramsay, T., Pauzé, E., Bagnato, M., and Potvin Kent, M. (2023). The impact of characters like Tony the Tiger and other child-targeted techniques used in food and beverage marketing. *Frontiers in Nutrition, 10.*

4 **Food companies run:** Fazzino, T. L. (2022). The reinforcing natures of hyper-palatable foods: Behavioral evidence for their reinforcing properties and the role of the US food industry in promoting their availability. *Current Addiction Reports*, *9*(4), 298–306. https://doi.org/10.1007/s40429-022-00417-8; Fazzino, T. L., Rohde, K., and Sullivan, D. K. (2019). Hyper-palatable foods: Development of a quantitative definition and application to the US food system database. *Obesity*, *27*(11), 1761–1768. https://doi.org/10.1002/oby.22639; Moss, M. (2014). *Salt, Sugar, Fat: How the Food Giants Hooked Us*. Random House.

5 **In the United States:** Williams, A. M., Couch, C. A., Emmerich, S. D., and Ogburn, D. F. (2025). Ultra-processed food consumption in youth and adults: United States, August 2021–August 2023. *NCHS Data Brief*, *536*. https://doi.org/10.15620/CDC/174612.

5 **These foods tend to be:** Calcaterra, V., Cena, H., Rossi, V., Santero, S., Bianchi, A., and Zuccotti, G. (2023). Ultra-processed food, reward system and childhood obesity. *Children*, *10*(5). https://doi.org/10.3390/children10050804; Lauria, F., Dello Russo, M., Formisano, A., et al. (2021). Ultra-processed foods consumption and diet quality of European children, adolescents and adults: Results from the I.Family study. *Nutrition, Metabolism and Cardiovascular Diseases*, *31*(11), 3031–3043. https://doi.org/10.1016/j.numecd.2021.07.019.

5 **Beyond lacking nutrients:** Lane, M., Gamage, E., Du, S., et al. (2024). "Ultra-processed food exposure and adverse health outcomes: umbrella review of epidemiological meta-analyses." *BMJ*, 384:e077310.

5 **These factors also influence:** Calcaterra et al. (2023); Fazzino et al. (2019); Miraglia del Giudice, M., Dinardo, G., et al. (2025). Ultra-processed foods and respiratory and allergic diseases in childhood: Epidemiological evidence and mechanistic insights. *Nutrients*, *17*(20). https://doi.org/10.3390/NU17203269.

5 **the pleasure of eating:** Calcaterra et al. (2023); Fazzino et al. (2019); Hall, K. D., Ayuketah, A., Brychta, R., et al. (2019). Ultra-processed diets cause excess calorie intake and weight gain: An inpatient randomized controlled trial of ad libitum food intake. *Cell Metabolism*, *30*(1), 67. https://doi.org/10.1016/J.CMET.2019.05.008; Peters, K. Z., and Naneix, F. (2022). The role of dopamine and endocannabinoid systems in prefrontal cortex development: Adolescence as a critical period. *Frontiers in Neural Circuits*, *16*, 939235. https://doi.org/10.3389/FNCIR.2022.939235.

6 **while different children:** Lauria et al. (2021).

6 **When kids internalize:** Butt, M., Harvey, A., Khesroh, E., Rigby, A., and Paul, I. M. (2023). Assessment and impact of paediatric internalized weight bias: A systematic review. *Pediatric Obesity*, *18*(7). https://doi.org/10.1111/ijpo.13040; Foster, T., Eaton, M., and Probst, Y. (2024). The relationship between internalised weight bias and biopsychosocial outcomes in children and youth: A systematic review. *Journal of Eating Disorders*, *12*(1), 38. https://doi.org/10.1186/s40337-023-00959-w; Spiel, E. C., Paxton, S.

J., and Yager, Z. (2012). Weight attitudes in 3- to 5-year-old children: Age differences and cross-sectional predictors. *Body Image*, *9*(4), 524–527.

6 **Some children show bias:** Musher-Eizenman, D. R., Holub, S. C., Miller, A. B., Goldstein, S. E., and Edwards-Leeper, L. (2004). Body size stigmatization in preschool children: The role of control attributions. *Journal of Pediatric Psychology*, *29*(8), 613–620. https://doi.org/10.1093/jpepsy/jsh063; Ruffman, T., O'Brien, K. S., Taumoepeau, M., Latner, J. D., and Hunter, J. A. (2016). Toddlers' bias to look at average versus obese figures relates to maternal anti-fat prejudice. *Journal of Experimental Child Psychology*, *142*, 195–202. https://doi.org/10.1016/J.JECP.2015.10.008; Spiel et al. (2012); Spiel, E. C., Rodgers, R. F., Paxton, S. J., et al. (2016). "He's got his father's bias": Parental influence on weight bias in young children. *British Journal of Developmental Psychology*, *34*(2), 198–211; Winograd, D., Goldschmidt, A. B., and Lydecker, J. (2024). Associations among parents' internalized weight bias, negative child-focused body talk, and feeding behaviors. *Eating Behaviors*, *52*, 101848. https://doi.org/10.1016/j.eatbeh.2024.101848.

6 **They often turn:** Foster et al. (2024).

6 **more likely to develop:** Butt et al. (2023); Gmeiner, M. S., and Warschburger, P. (2020). Intrapersonal predictors of weight bias internalization among elementary school children: a prospective analysis. *BMC Pediatrics*, *20*(1), 408. https://doi.org/10.1186/s12887-020-02264-w; Paxton, S. J., and Damiano, S. R. (2017). The development of body image and weight bias in childhood. *Advances in Child Development and Behavior*, *52*, 269–298. https://doi.org/10.1016/bs.acdb.2016.10.006; Tatangelo, G., McCabe, M., Mellor, D., and Mealey, A. (2016). A systematic review of body dissatisfaction and sociocultural messages related to the body among preschool children. *Body Image*, *18*, 86–95. https://doi.org/10.1016/J.BODYIM.2016.06.003; Zancu, A. S., and Diaconu-Gherasim, L. R. (2024). Weight stigma and mental health outcomes in early-adolescents. The mediating role of internalized weight bias and body esteem. *Appetite*, *196*, 107276. https://doi.org/10.1016/j.appet.2024.107276.

6 **Weight stigma doesn't:** Braddock, A., Browne, N. T., Houser, M., Blair, G., and Williams, D. R. (2023). Weight stigma and bias: A guide for pediatric clinicians. *Obesity Pillars*, *6*, 100058. https://doi.org/10.1016/J.OBPILL.2023.100058; Fields, L. C., Brown, C., Skelton, J. A., Cain, K. S., and Cohen, G. M. (2021). Internalized weight bias, teasing, and self-esteem in children with overweight or obesity. *Childhood Obesity (Print)*, *17*(1), 43–50. https://doi.org/10.1089/chi.2020.0150; Ozbardakci, E. V., and Lydecker, J. A. (2023). Reframing how providers advocate for adolescent well-being in body image, eating, and weight. *Journal of the American Academy of Child and Adolescent Psychiatry*, *62*(9), 957–962. https://doi.org/10.1016/j.jaac.2023.03.008; Palad, C. J., Yarlagadda, S., and Stanford, F. C. (2019). Weight stigma and its impact on paediatric care. *Current Opinion in Endocrinology, Diabetes and Obesity*, *26*(1), 19–24. https://doi.org/10.1097/MED.0000000000000453; Paxton and Damiano (2017);

Spiel et al. (2016); Pudney, E. V., Himmelstein, M. S., and Puhl, R. M. (2019). The role of weight stigma in parental weight talk. *Pediatric Obesity*, *14*(10), e12534. https://doi.org/10.1111/ijpo.12534.

6 **The weight-management industry:** Allied Market Research. (2021). *Weight Loss and Weight Management Diet Market Size, Share & Trends*. Retrieved July 19, 2023, from https://www.alliedmarketresearch.com/weight-loss-management-diet-market.

6 **availability of GLP-1 inhibitors:** Morris, H., and King, J. (2024, February). *GLP-1s: More than just obesity drugs*. J.P.Morgan Asset Management. https://am.jpmorgan.com/us/en/asset-management/adv/insights/portfolio-insights/equity/glp-1s-more-than-just-obesity-drugs/; Hampl, S. E., Hassink, S. G., Skinner, A. C., et al. (2023). *Clinical Practice Guideline for the Evaluation and Treatment of Children and Adolescents with Obesity*. http://publications.aap.org/pediatrics/article-pdf/151/2/e2022060640/1440824/peds_2022060640.pdf.

6 **we've seen an uptick:** Perng, W., Conway, R., Mayer-Davis, E., and Dabelea, D. (2023). Youth-onset type 2 diabetes: The epidemiology of an awakening epidemic. *Diabetes Care*, *46*(3), 490–499. https://doi.org/10.2337/dci22-0046; Ruan, X., Zhu, A., Wang, T., et al. (2025). Global prevalence of hypertension in children and adolescents younger than 19 years: A systematic review and meta-analysis. *JAMA Pediatrics*, *179*(9), 987–999. https://doi.org/10.1001/JAMAPEDIATRICS.2025.2206; Tönnies, T., Brinks, R., Isom, S., et al. (2022). Projections of type 1 and type 2 diabetes burden in the U.S. population aged 20 years through 2060: The SEARCH for diabetes in youth study. *Diabetes Care*, *46*(2), 313–320. https://doi.org/10.2337/dc22-0945.

7 **They will require governmental:** Alfraidi, A., Alafif, N., and Alsukait, R. (2023). The impact of mandatory food-marketing regulations on purchase and exposure: A narrative review. *Children*, *10*(8), 1277. https://doi.org/10.3390/children10081277; Global Food Research Program at UNC–Chapel Hill, 2022; Lafontaine, J., Hanson, I., and Wild, C. (2025). The impact of the social media industry as a commercial determinant of health on the digital food environment for children and adolescents: A scoping review. *BMJ Global Health*, *10*(2), e014667. https://doi.org/10.1136/BMJGH-2023-014667; Sing, F., Mackay, S., Swinburn, B., and Garton, K. (2025). A political economy analysis of the legislative response to unhealthy food and beverage marketing in Chile, Canada and the UK. *Globalization and Health*, *21*(1). https://doi.org/10.1186/s12992-024-01093-1; World Health Organization. (2023). *Policies to protect children from the harmful impact of food marketing WHO guideline*; Wilking, C., Moukalled, S., and Polacsek, M. (2023). Reducing student exposure to digital food and beverage marketing: Policy and practice recommendations. *Journal of School Health*, *93*(7), 638–643. https://doi.org/10.1111/josh.13315.

7 **including one to reduce:** Jensen et al. (2022).

1: Feed with Curiosity

22 **studies observe fathers:** Davison, K. K., Haines, J., Garcia, E. A., Douglas, S., and McBride, B. (2020). Fathers' food parenting: A scoping review of the literature from 1990 to 2019. *Pediatric Obesity, 15*(10). https://doi.org/10.1111/ijpo.12654; De-Jongh González, O., Tugault-Lafleur, C. N., O'Connor, T. M., Hughes, S. O., and Mâsse, L. C. (2021). Are fathers' and mothers' food parenting practices differentially associated with children's eating behaviors? *Appetite, 166*. https://doi.org/10.1016/j.appet.2021.105434; Fielding-Singh, P. (2017). Dining with dad: Fathers' influences on family food practices. *Appetite, 117*, 98–108. https://doi.org/10.1016/j.appet.2017.06.013; Frankel, L. A., and Kuno, C. B. (2019). The moderating role of parent gender on the relationship between restrictive feeding and a child's self-regulation in eating: Results from mother-only samples may not apply to both parents. *Appetite, 143*. https://doi.org/10.1016/j.appet.2019.104424; Gevers, D. W. M., van Assema, P., Sleddens, E. F. C., de Vries, N. K., and Kremers, S. P. J. (2015). Associations between general parenting, restrictive snacking rules, and adolescent's snack intake. The roles of fathers and mothers and interparental congruence. *Appetite, 87*, 184–191. https://doi.org/10.1016/J.APPET.2014.12.220; Khandpur, N., Charles, J., Blaine, R. E., Blake, C., and Davison, K. (2016). Diversity in fathers' food parenting practices: A qualitative exploration within a heterogeneous sample. *Appetite, 101*, 134–145. https://doi.org/10.1016/j.appet.2016.02.161; Pratt, M., Hoffmann, D., Taylor, M., and Musher-Eizenman, D. (2019). Structure, coercive control, and autonomy promotion: A comparison of fathers' and mothers' food parenting strategies. *Journal of Health Psychology, 24*(13), 1863–1877. https://doi.org/10.1177/1359105317707257; Walton, K., Haycraft, E., Jewell, K., Breen, A., Simpson, J. R., and Haines, J. (2019). The family mealtime observation study (FaMOS): Exploring the role of family functioning in the association between mothers' and fathers' food parenting practices and children's nutrition risk. *Nutrients, 11*(3). https://doi.org/10.3390/nu11030630.

23 **certain strategies parents use:** Almaatani, D., Cory, E., Gardner, J., et al. (2023). Child and maternal factors associated with feeding practices in children with poor growth. *Nutrients, 15*(22), 4850. https://doi.org/10.3390/nu15224850; Baker, L. N., Witherspoon, D. O., Nicholson, J. S., and Fuglestad, A. J. (2023). The roles of child temperament, parent stress, and parenting style in family mealtimes. *Appetite, 188*. https://doi.org/10.1016/j.appet.2023.106758; Berge, J. M., Miller, J., Veblen-Mortenson, S., Kunin-Batson, A., Sherwood, N. E., and French, S. A. (2020). A bidirectional analysis of feeding practices and eating behaviors in parent/child dyads from low-income and minority households. *Journal of Pediatrics, 221*, 93. https://doi.org/10.1016/J.JPEDS.2020.02.001; Bergmeier, H., Skouteris, H., Horwood, S., Hooley, M., and Richardson, B. (2014). Associations between child temperament, maternal feeding practices and child body mass index during the preschool years: A systematic review of

the literature. *Obesity Reviews*, *15*(1), 9–18. https://doi.org/10.1111/OBR.12066; Messerli-Bürgy, N., Stülb, K., Kakebeeke, T. H., et al. (2018). Emotional eating is related with temperament but not with stress biomarkers in preschool children. *Appetite*, *120*, 256–264. https://doi.org/10.1016/J.APPET.2017.08.032; Rendall, S., Dodd, H., and Harvey, K. (2022). Controlling feeding practices moderate the relationship between emotionality and food fussiness in young children. *Appetite*, *178*. https://doi.org/10.1016/J.APPET.2022.106259; Ruggiero, C. F., Hohman, E. E., Birch, L. L., Paul, I. M., and Savage, J. S. (2021). INSIGHT responsive parenting intervention effects on child appetite and maternal feeding practices through age 3 years. *Appetite*, *159*, 105060. https://doi.org/10.1016/J.APPET.2020.105060; Tauriello, S., Moding, K., Aronoff, N., Kubiniec, E., and Anzman-Frasca, S. (2023). Examining links between child temperament and feeding, eating, and weight outcomes: An updated systematic review of the literature. *Eating Behaviors*, 49. https://doi.org/10.1016/j.eatbeh.2023.101739.

23 **structured and supportive feeding:** Ju, S., Iwinski, S., and Bost, K. K. (2024). Temperament and emotional overeating: The mediating role of caregiver response to children's negative emotions. *Frontiers in Psychology*, *15*. https://www.frontiersin.org/journals/psychology/articles/10.3389/fpsyg.2024.1369252; Krupsky, K. L., Zvara, B. J., Khalsa, A. S., Andridge, R., Keim, S. A., and Anderson, S. E. (2024). Household chaos, child temperament, and structure-related feeding practices in toddlerhood: A moderation analysis. *Eating Behaviors*, *52*, 101838. https://doi.org/10.1016/J.EATBEH.2023.101838; Tauriello et al. (2023); Zimmer-Gembeck, M. J., McKay, A., and Webb, H. J. (2019). The food-related parenting context: Associations with parent mindfulness and children's temperament. *Mindfulness*, *10*(11), 2415–2428. https://doi.org/10.1007/S12671-019-01219-2/METRICS.

23 **if a child can self-regulate:** Edwards, K. L., Pickard, A., Farrow, C., et al. (2024). Differences in parental behaviour, emotions, and cognitions and between children's eating profiles. *Appetite*, *202*. https://doi.org/10.1016/J.APPET.2024.107641.

23 **whether a parent's feeding choices:** Burnett, A. J., Russell, C. G., Lacy, K. E., Worsley, A., and Spence, A. C. (2023). Mothers' descriptions of their feeding strategies in response to fussy eating with children of different levels of trait fussiness. *Appetite*, *187*. https://doi.org/10.1016/J.APPET.2023.106581; Finistrella, V., Gianni, N., Fintini, D., et al. (2024). Neophobia, sensory experience and child's schemata contribute to food choices. *Eating and Weight Disorders*, *29*(1), 25. https://doi.org/10.1007/S40519-024-01657-5; Savard, C., Bégin, S., and Gingras, V. (2022). Factors associated with eating in the absence of hunger among children and adolescents: A systematic review. *Nutrients*, *14*(22). https://doi.org/10.3390/nu14224715; Kininmonth, A. R., Herle, M., Haycraft, E., et al. (2023). Reciprocal associations between parental feeding practices and child eating behaviours from toddlerhood to early childhood: Bivariate latent change

analysis in the Gemini cohort. *Journal of Child Psychology and Psychiatry*, *64*(10), 1432–1445. https://doi.org/10.1111/JCPP.13819.

23 **Perhaps we should be using:** Cummings, J. R., Lipsky, L. M., Faith, M. S., and Nansel, T. R. (2024). Associations of appetitive traits and parental feeding style with diet quality during early childhood. *Journal of the Academy of Nutrition and Dietetics*. https://doi.org/10.1016/J.JAND.2024.02.004.

2: Eat with Embodied Independence

33 **Embodiment also describes what happens:** McBride, H., and Kwee, J. (2019). *Embodiment and Eating Disorders: Theory, Research, Prevention, and Treatment*. Routledge.

34 **Embodiment also helps protect:** Levine, M. P., and Smolak, L. (2016). The role of protective factors in the prevention of negative body image and disordered eating. *Eating Disorders*, *24*(1), 39–46. https://doi.org/10.1080/10640266.2015.1113826; McBride and Kwee (2019); Perey, I., and Cook-Cottone, C. (2020). Eating disorders, embodiment, and yoga: A conceptual overview. *Eating Disorders*, *28*(4), 315–329. https://doi.org/10.1080/10640266.2020.1771167.

34 **A child or an adult:** Chaves, E., Jeffrey, D. T., and Williams, D. R. (2023). Disordered eating and eating disorders in pediatric obesity: Assessment and next steps. *International Journal of Environmental Research and Public Health*, *20*(17), 6638. https://doi.org/10.3390/ijerph20176638.

34 **Avoidant/restrictive feeding:** Hog, L., and Dinkler, L. (2025). Recent insights into the epidemiology of avoidant/restrictive food intake disorder (ARFID). *Current Opinion in Psychiatry*. https://doi.org/10.1097/YCO.0000000000001041.

35 **Genetics, the gut microbiome:** Barakat, S., McLean, S. A., Bryant, E., et al. (2023). Risk factors for eating disorders: Findings from a rapid review. *Journal of Eating Disorders*, *11*(1). https://doi.org/10.1186/S40337-022-00717-4; Levine, M. P., and Sadeh-Sharvit, S. (2023). Preventing eating disorders and disordered eating in genetically vulnerable, high-risk families. *International Journal of Eating Disorders*, *56*(3), 523–534. https://doi.org/10.1002/EAT.23887.

36 **Media is one of the:** Blanchard, L., Conway-Moore, K., Aguiar, A. et al. (2023). Associations between social media, adolescent mental health, and diet: A systematic review. *Obesity Reviews*, *24*(S2), e13631. https://doi.org/10.1111/obr.13631; McBride and Kwee (2019).

37 **can start as early as preschool:** Herdzina, J., and Lauricella, A. R. (2020). *Media Literacy in Early Childhood Report Framework, Child Development Guidelines, and Tips for Implementation*. Erikson Institute.

38 **promote the ideology:** Ngqangashe, Y., Cullerton, K., Phulkerd, S., Huckel Schneider, C., Thow, A. M., and Friel, S. (2022). Discursive framing in policies for restricting the marketing of food and non-alcoholic beverages. *Food Policy*, *109*, 102270. https://doi.org/10.1016/J.FOODPOL.2022.102270; Westbury, S., Oyebode, O., van Rens, T., and Barber, T. M.

(2023). Obesity stigma: Causes, consequences, and potential solutions. *Current Obesity Reports*, *12*(1), 10. https://doi.org/10.1007/S13679-023-00495-3.

38 **weight and wellness:** Hampl, S. E., Hassink, S. G., Skinner, A. C., et al. (2023). *Clinical Practice Guideline for the Evaluation and Treatment of Children and Adolescents with Obesity.* http://publications.aap.org/pediatrics/article-pdf/151/2/e2022060640/1440824/peds_2022060640.pdf.; Safaei, M., Sundararajan, E. A., Driss, M., Boulila, W., and Shapi'i, A. (2021). A systematic literature review on obesity: Understanding the causes and consequences of obesity and reviewing various machine learning approaches used to predict obesity. *Computers in Biology and Medicine*, *136*. https://doi.org/10.1016/J.COMPBIOMED.2021.104754.

38 **even if research:** World Health Organization. (2023). *Policies to protect children from the harmful impact of food marketing.*

38 **This also perpetuates:** Bognar, G. (2020). The mismarriage of personal responsibility and health. *Cambridge Quarterly of Healthcare Ethics: CQ: The International Journal of Healthcare Ethics Committees*, *29*(2), 196–204. https://doi.org/10.1017/S0963180119000999; Hook, C. J., and Rose Markus, H. (2020). Health in the United States: Are appeals to choice and personal responsibility making Americans sick? *Perspectives on Psychological Science: A Journal of the Association for Psychological Science*, *15*(3), 643–664. https://doi.org/10.1177/1745691619896252.

38 **A parent openly dieting:** Barakat et al. (2023); Pudney, E. V, Himmelstein, M. S., and Puhl, R. M. (2019). The role of weight stigma in parental weight talk. *Pediatric Obesity*, *14*(10), e12534. https://doi.org/10.1111/ijpo.12534; Spiel, E. C., Rodgers, R. F., Paxton, S. J., et al. (2016). "He's got his father's bias": Parental influence on weight bias in young children. *British Journal of Developmental Psychology*, *34*(2), 198–211. https://doi.org/10.1111/bjdp.12123; Winograd, D., Goldschmidt, A. B., and Lydecker, J. (2024). Associations among parents' internalized weight bias, negative child-focused body talk, and feeding behaviors. *Eating Behaviors*, *52*, 101848. https://doi.org/10.1016/j.eatbeh.2024.101848.

39 **successful eating disorder prevention:** Ciao, A. C., Loth, K., and Neumark-Sztainer, D. (2014). Preventing eating disorder pathology: Common and unique features of successful eating disorders prevention programs. *Current Psychiatry Reports*, *16*(7). https://doi.org/10.1007/s11920-014-0453-0; Levine, M. P., and Smolak, L. (2016). The role of protective factors in the prevention of negative body image and disordered eating. *Eating Disorders*, *24*(1), 39–46. https://doi.org/10.1080/10640266.2015.1113826.

41 **Phrases like these:** Black, M. M., and Aboud, F. E. (2011). Responsive feeding is embedded in a theoretical framework of responsive parenting. *Journal of Nutrition*, *141*(3), 490–494. https://doi.org/10.3945/jn.110.129973.

43 **Exposing children to:** Balantekin, K. N., Anzman-Frasca, S., Francis, L. A., Ventura, A. K., Fisher, J. O., and Johnson, S. L. (2020). Positive parent-

ing approaches and their association with child eating and weight: A narrative review from infancy to adolescence. *Pediatric Obesity*, *15*(10). https://doi.org/10.1111/ijpo.12722; Fries, L. R., and Van Der Horst, K. (2019). Parental feeding practices and associations with children's food acceptance and picky eating. *Nestle Nutrition Institute Workshop Series*, 91, 31–39. https://doi.org/10.1159/000493676.

44 **This approach will look different:** Balantekin et al. (2020).

44 **distractions such as screens:** Kasper, N., Ball, S. C., Halverson, K., et al. (2019). Deconstructing the family meal: Are characteristics of the mealtime environment associated with the healthfulness of meals served? *Journal of the Academy of Nutrition and Dietetics*, *119*(8), 1296–1304. https://doi.org/10.1016/J.JAND.2019.01.009; Snuggs, S., and Harvey, K. (2023). Family mealtimes: A systematic umbrella review of characteristics, correlates, outcomes and interventions. *Nutrients*, *15*(13). https://doi.org/10.3390/nu15132841.

45 **consider that in 1977:** Piernas, C., and Popkin, B. M. (2010). Trends in snacking among U.S. children. *Health Affairs (Project Hope)*, *29*(3), 398. https://doi.org/10.1377/HLTHAFF.2009.0666.

45 **the average two-to-five-year-old:** Dunford, E. K. and Popkin, B. M. (2018). 37 year snacking trends for US children 1977–2014. *Pediatric Obesity*, *13*(4), 247–255. https://doi.org/10.1111/ijpo.12220.

45 **frequent eating:** Virkkala, V. F., Eloranta, A. M., Suominen, et al. (2023). Associations of diet quality, food consumption, eating frequency and eating behaviour with dental caries experience in Finnish children: A 2-year longitudinal study. *British Journal of Nutrition*, *129*(8), 1415–1425. https://doi.org/10.1017/S0007114522002550.

48 **the researchers ask so few questions:** Researchers use surveys to study different types of restriction, including the three most common types. First is overt restriction, when a parent restricts a child's food and the child knows they are being restricted. Researchers who study the effects of overt restriction ask questions like whether a parent limits how often a child can have sweets, snacks, "high fat" foods, "unhealthy" foods, or how much they are allowed to eat of them. Parents are also asked if they keep foods out of reach and sometimes whether they are restricting their kids for weight or health reasons. Second is *covert restriction*, when a parent restricts a child's food but the child *doesn't* know they are being restricted. To measure the effects of this method, researchers ask parents whether they avoid places where "unhealthy" foods are sold, avoid bringing sweets or other "unhealthy" foods into the house, or avoid eating "unhealthy" foods when their child is around to avoid exposing the child to them. Finally there is *limit setting*, when parents limit how often certain foods are made available to their child, sometimes restricting how much kids can eat, and the child is aware of it. This type of restriction has elements of covert and overt restriction, but unlike those two types, researchers don't have a standard set of questions they ask parents about it; Birch, L. L., Fisher, J. O., Grimm-Thomas, K., Markey,

C. N., Sawyer, R., and Johnson, S. L. (2001). "Confirmatory factor analysis of the Child Feeding Questionnaire: A measure of parental attitudes, beliefs and practices about child feeding and obesity proneness." *Appetite*, *36*(3), 201–210. https://doi.org/10.1006/appe.2001.0398; Yee, A. Z. H., Lwin, M. O., and Ho, S. S. (2017). The influence of parental practices on child promotive and preventive food consumption behaviors: A systematic review and meta-analysis. *International Journal of Behavioral Nutrition and Physical Activity*, *14*(1), 47. https://doi.org/10.1186/s12966-017-0501-3; Ogden, J., Reynolds, R., and Smith, A. (2006). "Expanding the concept of parental control: A role for overt and covert control in children's snacking behaviour?" *Appetite*, *47*(1), 100–106. https://doi.org/10.1016/j.appet.2006.03.330; Say, A., de la Piedad Garcia, X., and Mallan, K. M. (2023). The correlation between different operationalisations of parental restrictive feeding practices and children's eating behaviours: Systematic review and meta-analyses. *Appetite*, *180*. https://doi.org/10.1016/j.appet.2022.106320.

49 **One group of researchers:** Berge, J. M., Miller, J., Veblen-Mortenson, S., Kunin-Batson, A., Sherwood, N. E., and French, S. A. (2020). A bidirectional analysis of feeding practices and eating behaviors in parent/child dyads from low-income and minority households. *Journal of Pediatrics*, *221*, 93. https://doi.org/10.1016/J.JPEDS.2020.02.001.

49 **It's unclear whether restriction:** Durão, C., Andreozzi, V., Oliveira, A., et al. (2015). Maternal child-feeding practices and dietary inadequacy of 4-year-old children. *Appetite*, *92*, 15–23. https://doi.org/10.1016/j.appet.2015.04.067; Werner, L. M., and Mallan, K. M. (2024). Associations between restrictive feeding practices and children's dietary intake: Systematic review and meta-analyses. *Appetite*, *200*. https://doi.org/10.1016/j.appet.2024.107508.

49 **Some researchers have:** Boots, S. B., Tiggemann, M., and Corsini, N. (2018). "That's enough now!": A prospective study of the effects of maternal control on children's snack intake. *Appetite*, *126*, 1–7. https://doi.org/10.1016/j.appet.2018.03.008; Gevers, D. W. M., van Assema, P., Sleddens, E. F. C., de Vries, N. K., and Kremers, S. P. J. (2015). Associations between general parenting, restrictive snacking rules, and adolescent's snack intake. The roles of fathers and mothers and interparental congruence. *Appetite*, *87*, 184–191. https://doi.org/10.1016/J.APPET.2014.12.220; Mason, T. B. (2024). Interactions of parental feeding characteristics and adolescent emotional eating in relation to unhealthful food and sugar-sweetened beverage intake among adolescents. *Appetite*, *193*. https://doi.org/10.1016/j.appet.2023.107125; Mueller, C., Zeinstra, G. G., Forde, C. G., and Jager, G. (2024). Sweet rules: Parental restriction linked to lower free sugar and higher fruit intake in 4–7-year-old children. *Food Quality and Preference*, 113. https://doi.org/10.1016/j.foodqual.2023.105071.

50 **observed that restricted kids:** Bauer, K. W., Haines, J., Miller, A. L., et al. (2017). Maternal restrictive feeding and eating in the absence of hunger among toddlers: A cohort study. *International Journal of Behavioral Nutri-*

tion and Physical Activity, *14*(1). https://doi.org/10.1186/s12966-017-0630-8; Berge et al. (2020); Binder, A., Naderer, B., and Matthes, J. (2020a). A "forbidden fruit effect": An eye-tracking study on children's visual attention to food marketing. *International Journal of Environmental Research and Public Health*, *17*(6). https://doi.org/10.3390/ijerph17061859; Blaine, R. E., Kachurak, A., Davison, K. K., Klabunde, R., and Fisher, J. O. (2017). Food parenting and child snacking: A systematic review. *International Journal of Behavioral Nutrition and Physical Activity*, *14*(1), 146. https://doi.org/10.1186/s12966-017-0593-9; Derks, I. P. M., Bolhuis, K., Sijbrands, E. J. G., Gaillard, R., Hillegers, M. H. J., and Jansen, P. W. (2019). Predictors and patterns of eating behaviors across childhood: Results from the Generation R study. *Appetite*, *141*. https://doi.org/10.1016/j.appet.2019.05.026; Fisher, J. O. and Birch, L. L. (1999). Restricting access to palatable foods affects children's behavioral response, food selection, and intake. *American Journal of Clinical Nutrition*, *69*(6), 1264–1272. https://doi.org/10.1093/AJCN/69.6.1264; Say et al. (2023); Tan, C. C., Ruhl, H., Chow, C. M., and Ellis, L. (2016). Retrospective reports of parental feeding practices and emotional eating in adulthood: The role of food preoccupation. *Appetite*, *105*, 410–415. https://doi.org/10.1016/J.APPET.2016.06.009; Webber, L., Cooke, L., Hill, C., and Wardle, J. (2010). Associations between children's appetitive traits and maternal feeding practices. *Journal of the American Dietetic Association*, *110*(11), 1718–1722. https://doi.org/10.1016/j.jada.2010.08.007.

50 **Some have even observed:** Jennings, K. M., Loth, K. A., Tate, A. D., Miner, M. H., and Berge, J. M. (2019). Application of latent profile analysis to define subgroups of parenting styles and food parenting practices. *Appetite*, *139*, 8–18. https://doi.org/10.1016/j.appet.2019.04.001; Norman, J., Kelly, B., McMahon, A. T., et al. (2018). Children's self-regulation of eating provides no defense against television and online food marketing. *Appetite*, *125*, 438–444. https://doi.org/10.1016/j.appet.2018.02.026.

50 **including genetics and temperament:** Bergmeier, H., Skouteris, H., Horwood, S., Hooley, M., and Richardson, B. (2014). Associations between child temperament, maternal feeding practices and child body mass index during the preschool years: A systematic review of the literature. *Obesity Reviews*, *15*(1), 9–18. https://doi.org/10.1111/OBR.12066; Farrow, C. V., Haycraft, E., and Blissett, J. M. (2015). Teaching our children when to eat: How parental feeding practices inform the development of emotional eating—a longitudinal experimental design. *American Journal of Clinical Nutrition*, *101*(5), 908–913. https://doi.org/10.3945/ajcn.114.103713; Gouveia, M. J., Canavarro, M. C., and Moreira, H. (2019). How can mindful parenting be related to emotional eating and overeating in childhood and adolescence? The mediating role of parenting stress and parental child-feeding practices. *Appetite*, *138*, 102–114. https://doi.org/10.1016/J.APPET.2019.03.021; Jansen, E., Mulkens, S., and Jansen, A. (2007). Do not eat the red food!: Prohibition of snacks leads

to their relatively higher consumption in children. *Appetite*, *49*(3), 572–577. https://doi.org/10.1016/j.appet.2007.03.229; Lansigan, R. K., Emond, J. A., and Gilbert-Diamond, D. (2014). Understanding eating in the absence of hunger among young children: A systematic review of existing studies. *Appetite*, *85*, 36–47. https://doi.org/10.1016/J.APPET.2014.10.032; Philippe, K., Chabanet, C., Issanchou, S., and Monnery-Patris, S. (2021). Young children's eating in the absence of hunger: Links with child inhibitory control, child BMI, and maternal controlling feeding practices. *Frontiers in Psychology*, *12*. https://doi.org/10.3389/fpsyg.2021.653408; Renier, T. J., Yeum, D., Emond, J. A., et al. (2023). Elucidating pathways to pediatric obesity: A study evaluating obesity polygenic risk scores related to appetitive traits in children. *International Journal of Obesity*. https://doi.org/10.1038/s41366-023-01385-3; Riera-Navarro, C., and Nicklaus, S. (2025). Restrictive, but not instrumental feeding, is associated with eating in the absence of hunger in toddlers: A cross-sectional lab-based study. *Appetite*, *204*. https://doi.org/10.1016/j.appet.2024.107746; Rollins, B. Y., Loken, E., Savage, J. S., and Birch, L. L. (2014). Maternal controlling feeding practices and girls' inhibitory control interact to predict changes in BMI and eating in the absence of hunger from 5 to 7 y. *American Journal of Clinical Nutrition*, *99*(2), 249–257. https://doi.org/10.3945/AJCN.113.063545; Savard, C., Bégin, S., and Gingras, V. (2022). Factors associated with eating in the absence of hunger among children and adolescents: A systematic review. *Nutrients*, *14*(22). https://doi.org/10.3390/nu14224715.

50 **some researchers suspect:** Jansen et al. (2007).

50 **Psychological reactance:** Rosenberg, B., and Siegel, J. T. (2016). A 50-year review of psychological reactance theory: Do not read this article. *Psychology | Faculty Scholarship*, 3. https://doi.org/10.1037/mot0000091.

51 **the child might feel:** Riera-Navarro and Nicklaus (2025).

54 **having a parent who:** Barakat et al. (2023); Koreshe, E., Paxton, S., Miskovic-Wheatley, J., et al. (2023). Prevention and early intervention in eating disorders: Findings from a rapid review. *Journal of Eating Disorders*, *11*(1). https://doi.org/10.1186/s40337-023-00758-3.

54 **Most researchers studying restriction:** Francis, L. A., and Birch, L. L. (2005). Maternal influences on daughters' restrained eating behavior. *Health Psychology: Official Journal of the Division of Health Psychology, American Psychological Association*, *24*(6), 548. https://doi.org/10.1037/0278-6133.24.6.548; Gruber, M., König, D., Holzhäuser, J., et al. (2020). Parental feeding practices and the relationship with parents in female adolescents and young adults with eating disorders: A case control study. *PLOS One*, *15*(11), e0242518. https://doi.org/10.1371/JOURNAL.PONE.0242518; Harris, H. A., Kininmonth, A. R., Nas, Z., et al. (2024). Prospective associations between early childhood parental feeding practices and eating disorder symptoms and disordered eating behaviors in adolescence. *International Journal of Eating Disorders*, *57*(3), 716–726. https://doi.org/10.1002/eat.24159; Hazzard, V. M., Loth, K. A., Berge, J. M., Larson, N. I.,

Fulkerson, J. A., and Neumark-Sztainer, D. (2020). Does exposure to controlling parental feeding practices during adolescence predict disordered eating behaviors eight years later in emerging adulthood? *Pediatric Obesity*, *15*(10), e12709. https://doi.org/10.1111/IJPO.12709; Loth, K. A., Maclehose, R. F., Fulkerson, J. A., Crow, S., and Neumark-Sztainer, D. (2014). Are food restriction and pressure-to-eat parenting practices associated with adolescent disordered eating behaviors? *International Journal of Eating Disorders*, *47*(3), 310. https://doi.org/10.1002/EAT.22189; Moursi, M. M., Martin-Prével, Y., Eymard-Duvernay, S., et al. (2008). Assessment of child feeding practices using a summary index: Stability over time and association with child growth in urban Madagascar. *American Journal of Clinical Nutrition*, *87*(5), 1472–1479. https://doi.org/10.1093/AJCN/87.5.1472; Schmidt, R., Hiemisch, A., Kiess, W., and Hilbert, A. (2019). Interaction effects of child weight status and parental feeding practices on children's eating disorder symptomatology. *Nutrients*, *11*(10), 2433. https://doi.org/10.3390/NU11102433; Stromberg, S. E., Wheeler, P. B., Chardon, M. L., and Janicke, D. M. (2019). Parent perceptions of restrictive feeding on the relationship between youth BMI *z*-score and weight control behavior use in African American youth: A mediational study. *Eating Behaviors*, *33*, 67–72. https://doi.org/10.1016/j.eatbeh.2019.03.006.

54 **we know disordered eating:** Barakat et al. (2023); Bergmeier et al. (2014); Koreshe et al. (2023); Lansigan et al. (2014); Loth, K. A., Vomacka, E., Hazzard, V. M., Trofholz, A., and Berge, J. M. (2024). Associations between parental engagement in disordered eating behaviors and use of specific food parenting practices within a racially, ethnically, and socioeconomically diverse sample. *Appetite*, 107253. https://doi.org/10.1016/J.APPET.2024.107253; Miller, N., Mallan, K. M., Byrne, R., de Jersey, S., Jansen, E., and Daniels, L. A. (2020). Non-responsive feeding practices mediate the relationship between maternal and child obesogenic eating behaviours. *Appetite*, *151*. https://doi.org/10.1016/j.appet.2020.104648; Norton, L., Parkinson, J., Harris, N., and Hart, L. M. (2021). What factors predict the use of coercive food parenting practices among mothers of young children? An examination of food literacy, disordered eating and parent demographics. *International Journal of Environmental Research and Public Health*, *18*(19), 10538. https://doi.org/10.3390/ijerph181910538; Renier, T. J., Yeum, D., Emond, J. A., et al. (2023). Elucidating pathways to pediatric obesity: A study evaluating obesity polygenic risk scores related to appetitive traits in children. *International Journal of Obesity*. https://doi.org/10.1038/s41366-023-01385-3; Rollins, B. Y., Savage, J. S., Fisher, J. O., and Birch, L. L. (2016). Alternatives to restrictive feeding practices to promote self-regulation in childhood: A developmental perspective. *Pediatric Obesity*, *11*(5), 326–332. https://doi.org/10.1111/IJPO.12071; Ruzicka, E. B., Darling, K. E., Fahrenkamp, A. J., and Sato, A. F. (2018). Familial influences on the use of controlling feeding practices with adolescents. *Appetite*, *127*, 155–162. https://doi.org/10.1016/j.appet.2018.04.031; Savard

et al. (2022); Webb, H. J., and Haycraft, E. (2019). Parental body dissatisfaction and controlling child feeding practices: A prospective study of Australian parent-child dyads. *Eating Behaviors*, *32*, 1–6. https://doi.org/10.1016/J.EATBEH.2018.10.002.

54 **whether parents discuss their own:** Barakat et al. (2023); Koreshe et al. (2023).

55 **There's a tiny bit:** Fisher, J. O., and Birch, L. L. (2000). Parents' restrictive feeding practices are associated with young girls' negative self-evaluation of eating. *Journal of the American Dietetic Association*, *100*(11), 1341–1346. https://doi.org/10.1016/S0002-8223(00)00378-3; Oliveira, S., Marta-Simões, J., and Ferreira, C. (2019). Early parental eating messages and disordered eating: The role of body shame and inflexible eating. *Journal of Psychology*, *153*(6), 615–627. https://doi.org/10.1080/00223980.2019.1583162; Oliveira, S., Pires, C., and Ferreira, C. (2020). Does the recall of caregiver eating messages exacerbate the pathogenic impact of shame on eating and weight-related difficulties? *Eating and Weight Disorders*, *25*(2), 471–480. https://doi.org/10.1007/S40519-018-0625-8/METRICS; Puhl, R. M., and Schwartz, M. B. (2003). If you are good you can have a cookie: How memories of childhood food rules link to adult eating behaviors. *Eating Behaviors*, *4*(3), 283–293. https://doi.org/10.1016/S1471-0153(03)00024-2.

56 **kids who have been delayed:** Kaynak, Ö., Winters, K. C., Cacciola, J., Kirby, K. C., and Arria, A. M. (2014). Providing alcohol for underage youth: What messages should we be sending parents? *Journal of Studies on Alcohol and Drugs*, *75*(4), 590. https://doi.org/10.15288/JSAD.2014.75.590.

59 **these programs show promise:** Babbott, K. M., Consedine, N. S., and Roberts, M. (2024). Your body is your home: The feasibility of an intuitive eating intervention for early adolescents. *International Journal of Eating Disorders*. https://doi.org/10.1002/eat.24163.

59 **"just about right":** Dowling, M. L., Hubbard, M. E., and Agnihotri, R. (2024). Association of parent and child intuitive eating: A scoping review. *American Journal of Lifestyle Medicine*. https://doi.org/10.1177/15598276241279223.

61 **thinking in terms:** Melbye, E. L., and Hansen, H. (2015). Promotion and prevention focused feeding strategies: Exploring the effects on healthy and unhealthy child eating. *BioMed Research International*, 306306. https://doi.org/10.1155/2015/306306.

61 **restricted kids are more likely:** Boots, S. B., Tiggemann, M., Corsini, N., and Mattiske, J. (2015). Managing young children's snack food intake. The role of parenting style and feeding strategies. *Appetite*, *92*, 94–101. https://doi.org/10.1016/j.appet.2015.05.012; Yee, A. Z. H., Lwin, M. O., and Ho, S. S. (2017). The influence of parental practices on child promotive and preventive food consumption behaviors: A systematic review and meta-analysis. *International Journal of Behavioral Nutrition and Physical Activity*, *14*(1), 47. https://doi.org/10.1186/s12966-017-0501-3.

61 **fewer conflicts with:** Gevers, D. W. M., van Assema, P., Sleddens, E. F. C., de Vries, N. K., and Kremers, S. P. J. (2015). Associations between general parenting, restrictive snacking rules, and adolescent's snack intake. The roles of fathers and mothers and interparental congruence. *Appetite, 87*, 184–191. https://doi.org/10.1016/J.APPET.2014.12.220.

62 **boundaries that could more easily:** Rollins, B. Y., Savage, J. S., Fisher, J. O., and Birch, L. L. (2016). Alternatives to restrictive feeding practices to promote self-regulation in childhood: A developmental perspective. *Pediatric Obesity, 11*(5), 326–332. https://doi.org/10.1111/IJPO.12071.

63 **The way we model:** Jennings, K. M., Loth, K. A., Tate, A. D., Miner, M. H., and Berge, J. M. (2019). Application of latent profile analysis to define subgroups of parenting styles and food parenting practices. *Appetite, 139*, 8–18. https://doi.org/10.1016/j.appet.2019.04.001.

63 **the "structure":** Gregory, J. E., Paxton, S. J., and Brozovic, A. M. (2010). Pressure to eat and restriction are associated with child eating behaviours and maternal concern about child weight, but not child body mass index, in 2- to 4-year-old children. *Appetite, 54*(3), 550–556. https://doi.org/10.1016/j.appet.2010.02.013; Haines, J., Downing, K. L., Tang, L., Campbell, K. J., and Hesketh, K. D. (2018). Associations between maternal concern about child's weight and related behaviours and maternal weight-related parenting practices: A cross-sectional study. *International Journal of Behavioral Nutrition and Physical Activity, 15*(1). https://doi.org/10.1186/S12966-018-0738-5; Hyczko, A. V, Ruggiero, C. F., Hohman, et al. (2021). Sex differences in maternal restrictive feeding practices in the intervention nurses start infants growing on healthy trajectories study. *Academic Pediatrics, 21*(6); Loth, K. A., Mohamed, N., Trofholz, A., Tate, A., and Berge, J. M. (2021). Associations between parental perception of—and concern about—child weight and use of specific food-related parenting practices. *Appetite, 160*. https://doi.org/10.1016/j.appet.2020.105068; Robertson, M. D. A., Dempster, S., Doherty, L., and Sharpe, H. (2022). Exploring the association between parental anti-fat attitudes and restrictive feeding practices in a British and Irish sample. *Appetite, 168*. https://doi.org/10.1016/j.appet.2021.105755.

66 **Collaboration can reduce:** Kulis, E., Szczuka, Z., Banik, A., et al. (2025). Individual, dyadic, collaborative planning, physical activity, and nutrition: A randomized controlled trial in parent-child dyads. *Health Psychology: Official Journal of the Division of Health Psychology, American Psychological Association, 44*(2), 140–153. https://doi.org/10.1037/HEA0001405; Savage, J. S., Adams, E. L., Rollins, B. Y., Bleser, J. A., and Marini, M. E. (2020). Teaching families to manage intake of candy in the home: Results from a feasibility study using multiphase optimization strategy (MOST). *Obesity Science & Practice, 6*(6), 649. https://doi.org/10.1002/OSP4.446.

67 **implementing your limits:** Melbye and Hansen (2015).

68 **It's normal to:** Almaatani, D., Cory, E., Gardner, J., et al. (2023). Child and maternal factors associated with feeding practices in children with poor

growth. *Nutrients, 15*(22), 4850. https://doi.org/10.3390/nu15224850; Burnette, C. B., Hazzard, V. M., Linardon, J., Rodgers, R. F., Loth, K. A., and Neumark-Sztainer, D. (2023). How parental feeding practices relate to young people's intuitive eating: Cross-sectional and longitudinal associations by gender and weight concern. *Journal of Adolescent Health*, 73(6), 1145–1152. https://doi.org/10.1016/J.JADOHEALTH.2023.07.018; Jansen, E., Mallan, K. M., Nicholson, J. M., and Daniels, L. A. (2014). The feeding practices and structure questionnaire: Construction and initial validation in a sample of Australian first-time mothers and their 2-year olds. *International Journal of Behavioral Nutrition and Physical Activity*, *11*, 72. https://doi.org/10.1186/1479-5868-11-72; Kininmonth, A. R., Herle, M., Tommerup, K., et al. (2023). Parental feeding practices as a response to child appetitive traits in toddlerhood and early childhood: A discordant twin analysis of the Gemini cohort. *International Journal of Behavioral Nutrition and Physical Activity, 20*(1). https://doi.org/10.1186/S12966-023-01440-2; Taylor, C. M., and Emmett, P. M. (2019). Picky eating in children: Causes and consequences. *Proceedings of the Nutrition Society*, 78(2), 161–169. https://doi.org/10.1017/S0029665118002586; Wang, J., Zhu, B., Wu, R., Chang, Y. S., Cao, Y., and Zhu, D. (2022). Bidirectional associations between parental non-responsive feeding practices and child eating behaviors: A systematic review and meta-analysis of longitudinal prospective studies. *Nutrients, 14*(9). https://doi.org/10.3390/NU14091896.

68 **researchers studying pressure:** Barakat et al. (2023); Beckers, D., Karssen, L. T., Vink, J. M., Burk, W. J., and Larsen, J. K. (2021). Food parenting practices and children's weight outcomes: A systematic review of prospective studies. *Appetite, 158*, 105010. https://doi.org/10.1016/j.appet.2020.105010; Ellis, J. M., Schenk, R. R., Galloway, A. T., Zickgraf, H. F., Webb, R. M., and Martz, D. M. (2018). A multidimensional approach to understanding the potential risk factors and covariates of adult picky eating. *Appetite, 125*, 1–9. https://doi.org/10.1016/J.APPET.2018.01.016; Fries, L. R., and Van Der Horst, K. (2019). Parental feeding practices and associations with children's food acceptance and picky eating. *Nestle Nutrition Institute Workshop Series, 91*, 31–39. https://doi.org/10.1159/000493676; Grammer, A. C., Balantekin, K. N., Barch, D. M., Markson, L., and Wilfley, D. E. (2022). Parent-child influences on child eating self-regulation and weight in early childhood: A systematic review. *Appetite, 168*, 105733. https://doi.org/10.1016/J.APPET.2021.105733; Harris, H. A., Kininmonth, A. R., Nas, Z., et al. (2024). Prospective associations between early childhood parental feeding practices and eating disorder symptoms and disordered eating behaviors in adolescence. *International Journal of Eating Disorders*. https://doi.org/10.1002/eat.24159; Hazzard, V. M., Loth, K. A., Berge, J. M., Larson, N. I., Fulkerson, J. A., and Neumark-Sztainer, D. (2020). Does exposure to controlling parental feeding practices during adolescence predict disordered eating behaviors eight years later in emerging adulthood? *Pediatric Obesity, 15*(10), e12709. https://doi.org/10.1111/IJPO.12709; Houldcroft,

L., Farrow, C., and Haycraft, E. (2014). Perceptions of parental pressure to eat and eating behaviours in preadolescents: The mediating role of anxiety. *Appetite, 80*, 61–69. https://doi.org/10.1016/J.APPET.2014.05.002; Jansen, P. W., de Barse, L. M., Jaddoe, V. W. V., Verhulst, F. C., Franco, O. H., and Tiemeier, H. (2017). Bi-directional associations between child fussy eating and parents' pressure to eat: Who influences whom? *Physiology & Behavior, 176*, 101–106. https://doi.org/10.1016/J.PHYSBEH.2017.02.015; Loth et al. (2014); Małachowska, A., and Jeżewska-Zychowicz, M. (2023). Retrospective reports of parental feeding practices and current eating styles in Polish adults. *Nutrients, 15*(19). https://doi.org/10.3390/NU15194217; Webber, L., Cooke, L., Hill, C., and Wardle, J. (2010). Associations between children's appetitive traits and maternal feeding practices. *Journal of the American Dietetic Association, 110*(11), 1718–1722. https://doi.org/10.1016/j.jada.2010.08.007.

68 **A common misconception:** Ruzicka, E. B., Darling, K. E., and Sato, A. F. (2021). Controlling child feeding practices and child weight: A systematic review and meta-analysis. *Obesity Reviews: An Official Journal of the International Association for the Study of Obesity, 22*(3). https://doi.org/10.1111/OBR.13135.

68 **very little research:** Burnette et al. (2023); Dowling, M. L., Hubbard, M. E., and Agnihotri, R. (2024). Association of parent and child intuitive eating: A scoping review. *American Journal of Lifestyle Medicine.* https://doi.org/10.1177/15598276241279223.

69 **serve smaller portions:** Searle, B. R. E., Harris, H. A., Thorpe, K., and Jansen, E. (2020). What children bring to the table: The association of temperament and child fussy eating with maternal and paternal mealtime structure. *Appetite, 151.* https://doi.org/10.1016/J.APPET.2020.104680.

69 **Many studies have observed:** Barbosa, C., Lopes, C., Costa, A., Warkentin, S., and Oliveira, A. (2023). Parental child-feeding practices at 4 years of age are associated with dietary patterns of 7-year-olds. *Journal of Human Nutrition and Dietetics.* https://doi.org/10.1111/jhn.13151; Wang, J., Wei, X., Chang, Y. S., Hiyoshi, A., Winkley, K., and Cao, Y. (2022). The relationships between caregivers' concern about child weight and their nonresponsive feeding practices: A systematic review and meta-analysis. *Nutrients, 14*(14). https://doi.org/10.3390/NU14142885/S1; Yee et al. (2017).

69 ***how* you pressure:** Balantekin, K. N., Anzman-Frasca, S., Francis, L. A., Ventura, A. K., Fisher, J. O., and Johnson, S. L. (2020). Positive parenting approaches and their association with child eating and weight: A narrative review from infancy to adolescence. *Pediatric Obesity, 15*(10). https://doi.org/10.1111/ijpo.12722.

72 **many correlated factors:** Buja, A., Manfredi, M., Zampieri, C., et al. (2022). Is emotional eating associated with behavioral traits and Mediterranean diet in children? A cross-sectional study. *BMC Public Health, 22*(1). https://doi.org/10.1186/s12889-022-14192-8; Ju, S., Iwinski, S., and Bost, K. K. (2024). Temperament and emotional overeating: The mediating

role of caregiver response to children's negative emotions. *Frontiers in Psychology, 15.* https://www.frontiersin.org/journals/psychology/articles/10.3389/fpsyg.2024.1369252; Limbers, C. A., Greenwood, E., Shea, K., and Fergus, T. A. (2021). Metacognitive beliefs and emotional eating in adolescents. *Eating and Weight Disorders*, *26*(7), 2281–2286. https://doi.org/10.1007/s40519-020-01078-0; Shriver, L. H., Dollar, J. M., Calkins, S. D., Keane, S. P., Shanahan, L., and Wideman, L. (2021). Emotional eating in adolescence: effects of emotion regulation, weight status and negative body image. *Nutrients*, *13*(1), 1–12. https://doi.org/10.3390/nu13010079; Spinner, H., Thompson, K. A., Bauman, V., et al. (2024). Emotional dysregulation moderates the relation between perceived stress and emotional eating in adolescent military dependents. *International Journal of Eating Disorders*. https://doi.org/10.1002/eat.24217; Stone, R. A., Blissett, J., Haycraft, E., and Farrow, C. (2022). Predicting preschool children's emotional eating: The role of parents' emotional eating, feeding practices and child temperament. *Maternal and Child Nutrition*, *18*(3). https://doi.org/10.1111/mcn.13341.

72 **It may also be related:** Ju, S., Iwinski, S., Fiese, B. H., McBride, B. A., and Bost, K. K. (2022). Influences of child temperament and household chaos on preschoolers' emotional eating. *Childhood Obesity*, *18*(8), 523–532. https://doi.org/10.1089/chi.2021.0237; Stone et al. (2022); Vang, M., Sherrard, A., and Tan, C. C. (2023). Parents' emotion dysregulation and children's emotional overeating: The role of emotion regulation feeding. *Eating Behaviors*, *50*, 101795. https://doi.org/10.1016/J.EATBEH.2023.101795.

72 **We may be out:** Spinner et al. (2024).

72 **Using food for emotional regulation:** Pastore, M., Indrio, F., Bali, D., Vural, M., Giardino, I., and Pettoello-Mantovani, M. (2023). Alarming increase of eating disorders in children and adolescents. *Journal of Pediatrics*, *263*. https://doi.org/10.1016/j.jpeds.2023.113733; Tan et al. (2016).

73 **children with higher stress:** Henderson, K. A., Obeid, N., Buchholz, A., et al. (2022). Coping in adolescents: A mediator between stress and disordered eating. *Eating Behaviors*, 47. https://doi.org/10.1016/J.EATBEH.2022.101626.

73 **children who avoid:** Henderson et al. (2022).

3: Eat Together

82 **opportunities for us:** Brown, S. L., Teufel, J., Birch, D. A., and Abrams, T. E. (2019). Family meals and adolescent perceptions of parent–child connectedness. *Journal of Family Studies*, *25*(1), 34–45. https://doi.org/10.1080/13229400.2016.1200115.

82 **children in families that eat together:** Harbec, M.-J., and Pagani, L. S. (2018). Associations between early family meal environment quality and later well-being in school-age children. *Journal of Developmental and Behavioral Pediatrics*, *39*, 136–143; Harrison, M. L., Norris, N., Obeid, M., Fu, H., Weinstangel, M., and Sampson, M. E. (2015). Systematic review

of the effects of family meal frequency on psychosocial outcomes in youth. *Canadian Family Physician*, *61*; Snuggs, S. and Harvey, K. (2023). Family mealtimes: A systematic umbrella review of characteristics, correlates, outcomes and interventions. *Nutrients*, *15*(13). https://doi.org/10.3390/nu15132841; White, H. J., Haycraft, E., and Meyer, C. (2014). Family mealtimes and eating psychopathology: The role of anxiety and depression among adolescent girls and boys. *Appetite*, *75*, 173–179. https://doi.org/10.1016/J.APPET.2014.01.007.

82 **Parents who hold:** Utter, J., Larson, N., Berge, J. M., Eisenberg, M. E., Fulkerson, J. A., and Neumark-Sztainer, D. (2018). Family meals among parents: Associations with nutritional, social and emotional wellbeing. *Preventive Medicine*, *113*, 7–12. https://doi.org/10.1016/J.YPMED.2018.05.006.

82 **family meals may:** Utter et al. (2018).

83 **infants and toddlers:** Baker, L. N., Witherspoon, D. O., Nicholson, J. S., and Fuglestad, A. J. (2023). The roles of child temperament, parent stress, and parenting style in family mealtimes. *Appetite*, *188*. https://doi.org/10.1016/j.appet.2023.106758; Saltzman, J. A., Musaad, S., Bost, K. K., McBride, B. A., and Fiese, B. H. (2019). Associations between father availability, mealtime distractions and routines, and maternal feeding responsiveness: An observational study. *Journal of Family Psychology*, *33*(4), 465–475. https://doi.org/10.1037/fam0000519; Verhage, C. L., Gillebaart, M., van der Veek, S. M. C., and Vereijken, C. M. J. L. (2018). The relation between family meals and health of infants and toddlers: A review. *Appetite*, *127*, 97–109. https://doi.org/10.1016/J.APPET.2018.04.010.

83 **Kids who have family meals:** Bailey-Davis, L., Poulsen, M. N., Hirsch, A. G., Pollak, J., Glass, T. A., and Schwartz, B. S. (2017). Home food rules in relation to youth eating behaviors, body mass index, waist circumference, and percent body fat. *Journal of Adolescent Health*, *60*(3), 270–276. https://doi.org/10.1016/j.jadohealth.2016.09.020; Dallacker, M., Hertwig, R., and Mata, J. (2019). Quality matters: A meta-analysis on components of healthy family meals. *Health Psychology: Official Journal of the Division of Health Psychology, American Psychological Association*, *38*(12), 1137–1149. https://doi.org/10.1037/HEA0000801; Hammons, A. J., and Fiese, B. H. (2011). Is frequency of shared family meals related to the nutritional health of children and adolescents? *Pediatrics*, *127*(6). https://doi.org/10.1542/peds.2010-1440; Kasper, N., Ball, S. C., Halverson, K., et al. (2019). Deconstructing the family meal: Are characteristics of the mealtime environment associated with the healthfulness of meals served? *Journal of the Academy of Nutrition and Dietetics*, *119*(8), 1296–1304. https://doi.org/10.1016/J.JAND.2019.01.009; Mahmood, L., González-Gil, E. M., Schwarz, P., et al. (2022). Frequency of family meals and food consumption in families at high risk of type 2 diabetes: The Feel4Diabetes-study. *European Journal of Pediatrics*, *181*(6), 2523–2534. https://doi.org/10.1007/s00431-022-04445-4; Robson, S. M., McCullough, M. B., Rex, S., Munafò, M. R., and Taylor, G. (2020). Family meal frequency, diet,

and family functioning: A systematic review with meta-analyses. *Journal of Nutrition Education and Behavior*, *52*(5), 553–564. https://doi.org/10.1016/j.jneb.2019.12.012; Snuggs and Harvey (2023); Vejrup, K., Hillesund, E. R., Agnihotri, N., Helle, C., and Øverby, N. C. (2023). Diet in early life is related to child mental health and personality at 8 years: Findings from the Norwegian Mother, Father and Child Cohort Study (MoBa). *Nutrients*, *15*(1). https://doi.org/10.3390/nu15010243.

83 **parents who have frequent:** Utter et al. (2018).

83 **family meals are associated:** Verhage et al. (2018).

83 **have less disordered eating:** Berge, J. M., MacLehose, R. F., Loth, K. A., Eisenberg, M. E., Fulkerson, J. A., and Neumark-Sztainer, D. (2015). Parent-adolescent conversations about eating, physical activity and weight: Prevalence across sociodemographic characteristics and associations with adolescent weight and weight-related behaviors. *Journal of Behavioral Medicine*, *38*(1), 122–135. https://doi.org/10.1007/s10865-014-9584-3; Harrison et al. (2015); White et al. (2014).

85 **greater mental health:** Ardakani, A., Monroe-Lord, L., Wakefield, D., and Castor, C. (2023). Parenting styles, food parenting practices, family meals, and weight status of African American families. *International Journal of Environmental Research and Public Health*, *20*(2). https://doi.org/10.3390/ijerph20021382; Berge et al. (2015); Hammons and Fiese (2011); Harrison et al. (2015); Mahmood et al. (2022); Snuggs and Harvey (2023); Utter et al. (2018).

85 **when the TV is on:** Kasper et al. (2019); Snuggs and Harvey (2023).

86 **Fun can go a long way:** Berge et al. (2015); Snuggs and Harvey (2023); White et al. (2014).

86 **the family meal structure:** Harbec and Pagani (2018).

86 **if a family is not functioning well:** Berge et al. (2015).

87 **What you eat as the parent:** Dallacker, M., Hertwig, R., and Mata, J. (2019). Quality matters: A meta-analysis on components of healthy family meals. *Health Psychology : Official Journal of the Division of Health Psychology, American Psychological Association*, *38*(12), 1137–1149. https://doi.org/10.1037/HEA0000801.

87 **children ate more nutricious meals:** Mahmood, L., González-Gil, E. M., Schwarz, P., et al. (2022). Frequency of family meals and food consumption in families at high risk of type 2 diabetes: the Feel4Diabetes-study. *European Journal of Pediatrics*, *181*(6), 2523–2534. https://doi.org/10.1007/s00431-022-04445-4; Snuggs, S., and Harvey, K. (2023). Family mealtimes: A systematic umbrella review of characteristics, correlates, outcomes and interventions. *Nutrients*, 15(13). https://doi.org/10.3390/nu15132841.

87 **There are benefits:** Anderson, S. E., Must, A., Curtin, C., and Bandini, L. G. (2012). Meals in our household: Reliability and initial validation of a questionnaire to assess child mealtime behaviors and family mealtime environments. *Journal of the Academy of Nutrition and Dietetics*, *112*(2), 276–284. https://doi.org/10.1016/j.jada.2011.08.035.

87 **the one-bite rule can be a tool:** Holley, C. E., Haycraft, E., and Farrow, C. (2015). "Why don't you try it again?": A comparison of parent led, home

based interventions aimed at increasing children's consumption of a disliked vegetable. *Appetite*, *87*, 215–222. https://doi.org/10.1016/j.appet.2014.12.216; Nekitsing, C., Hetherington, M. M., and Blundell-Birtill, P. (2018). Developing healthy food preferences in preschool children through taste exposure, sensory learning, and nutrition education. *Current Obesity Reports*, 7(1), 60–67. https://doi.org/10.1007/s13679-018-0297-8.

87 **At least one experimental:** Thorsteinsdottir, S., Olafsdottir, A. S., Traustadottir, O. U., and Njardvik, U. (2023). Changes in anxiety following taste education intervention: Fussy eating children with and without neurodevelopmental disorders. *Nutrients*, *15*(22), 4783. https://doi.org/10.3390/nu15224783.

89 **rewarding with food:** Berge, J. M., Miller, J., Veblen-Mortenson, S., Kunin-Batson, A., Sherwood, N. E., and French, S. A. (2020). A bidirectional analysis of feeding practices and eating behaviors in parent/child dyads from low-income and minority households. *Journal of Pediatrics*, *221*, 93. https://doi.org/10.1016/J.JPEDS.2020.02.001; Jansen, E., Williams, K. E., Mallan, K. M., Nicholson, J. M., and Daniels, L. A. (2018). Bidirectional associations between mothers' feeding practices and child eating behaviours. *International Journal of Behavioral Nutrition and Physical Activity*, *15*(1). https://doi.org/10.1186/s12966-018-0644-x; Philippe, K., Chabanet, C., Issanchou, S., and Monnery-Patris, S. (2021). Young children's eating in the absence of hunger: Links with child inhibitory control, child BMI, and maternal controlling feeding practices. *Frontiers in Psychology*, 12. https://doi.org/10.3389/fpsyg.2021.653408; Spielvogel, I., Naderer, B., Binder, A., and Matthes, J. (2021). The forbidden reward. The emergence of parent-child conflicts about food over time and the influence of parents' communication strategies and feeding practices. *Frontiers in Public Health*, *8*. https://doi.org/10.3389/fpubh.2020.604702; Yee, A. Z. H., Lwin, M. O., and Ho, S. S. (2017). The influence of parental practices on child promotive and preventive food consumption behaviors: A systematic review and meta-analysis. *International Journal of Behavioral Nutrition and Physical Activity*, *14*(1), 47. https://doi.org/10.1186/s12966-017-0501-3.

89 **consider praise:** Cooke, L. J., Chambers, L. C., Añez, E. V., and Wardle, J. (2011). Facilitating or undermining? The effect of reward on food acceptance. A narrative review. *Appetite*, *57*(2), 493–497. https://doi.org/10.1016/j.appet.2011.06.016; Holley et al. (2015). Remington, A., Añez, E., Croker, H., Wardle, J., and Cooke, L. (2012). Increasing food acceptance in the home setting: A randomized controlled trial of parent-administered taste exposure with incentives. *American Journal of Clinical Nutrition*, *95*(1), 72–77. https://doi.org/10.3945/ajcn.111.024596; Yee et al. (2017).

4: Eat Without Judgment

93 **One research group looked:** Roach, E., Viechnicki, G. B., Retzloff, L. B., Davis-Kean, P., Lumeng, J. C., and Miller, A. L. (2017). Family food talk, child eating behavior, and maternal feeding practices. *Appetite*, *117*, 40–50. https://doi.org/10.1016/J.APPET.2017.06.001.

94 **Children's brains:** Lafraire, J., Rioux, C., Giboreau, A., and Picard, D. (2016). Food rejections in children: Cognitive and social/environmental factors involved in food neophobia and picky/fussy eating behavior. *Appetite*, *96*, 347–357. https://doi.org/10.1016/J.APPET.2015.09.008.

94 **They will learn:** Freedman, I., Eilam, B., and Gesser-Edelsburg, A. (2021). Young children's food-related knowledge: Kindergartners' free categorization of food items. *Journal of Nutrition Education and Behavior*, *53*(6), 524–530. https://doi.org/10.1016/J.JNEB.2020.12.007; Nguyen, S. P., and Murphy, G. L. (2003). An apple is more than just a fruit: Cross-classification in children's concepts. *Child Development*, *74*(6), 1783. https://doi.org/10.1046/J.1467-8624.2003.00638.

95 **Kids will also internalize:** Monnery-Patris, S., Marty, L., Bayer, F., Nicklaus, S., and Chambaron, S. (2016). Explicit and implicit tasks for assessing hedonic- versus nutrition-based attitudes towards food in French children. *Appetite*, *96*, 580–587. https://doi.org/10.1016/J.APPET.2015.10.026.

95 **people hold this belief:** Lakritz, C., Tournayre, L., Ouellet, M., et al. (2022). Sinful foods: Measuring implicit associations between food categories and moral attributes in anorexic, orthorexic, and healthy subjects. *Frontiers in Nutrition*, 9. https://doi.org/10.3389/fnut.2022.884003.

95 **To say foods are *good* or *bad*:** Vijaykumar, S., McNeill, A., and Simpson, J. (2021). Associations between conflicting nutrition information, nutrition confusion and backlash among consumers in the UK. *Public Health Nutrition*, *24*(5), 914–923. https://doi.org/10.1017/S1368980021000124.

96 **they were banned:** US Food and Drug Administration. (2023, December 14). *Revocation of Uses of Partially Hydrogenated Oils in Foods; Confirmation of Effective Date*. Federal Register. https://www.federalregister.gov/documents/2023/12/14/2023-27506/revocation-of-uses-of-partially-hydrogenated-oils-in-foods-confirmation-of-effective-date.

96 **inconsistencies from parents:** Spielvogel et al. (2021).

96 **This may be fine:** Lee, C., Nagler, R. H., and Wang, N. (2018). Source-specific exposure to contradictory nutrition information: Documenting prevalence and effects on adverse cognitive and behavioral outcomes. *Health Communication*, *33*(4), 453–461. https://doi.org/10.1080/10410236.2016.1278495.

96 **avoiding things like fruits:** Huang, Y., Edirisinghe, I., and Burton-Freeman, B. M. (2016). Low-income shoppers and fruit and vegetables: What do they think? *Nutrition Today*, *51*(5), 242–250. https://doi.org/10.1097/NT.0000000000000176; Rodman, S. O., Palmer, A. M., Zachary, D. A., Hopkins, L. C., and Surkan, P. J. (2014). "They just say organic food is healthier": Perceptions of healthy food among supermarket shoppers in southwest Baltimore. *Culture, Agriculture, Food and Environment*, *36*(2), 83–92. https://doi.org/10.1111/CUAG.12036.

97 **children with access to free school lunch:** Cohen, J., Gosliner, W., et al. (2023). Impact of Massachusetts' Healthy School Meals for All Policy on Families. Center for Health Innovation, Research, and Policy. https://healthyeatingresearch.org/research/impact-of-massachusetts-healthy-

school-meals-for-all-policy-on-families/; Domina, T., Clark, L., Radsky, V., and Bhaskar, R. (2024). There is such a thing as a free lunch: School meals, stigma, and student discipline. *American Educational Research Journal*, *61*(2), 287–327. https://doi.org/10.3102/00028312231222266.

97 **a long history of racism:** Fielding-Singh, P. (2021). *How the Other Half Eats*. Little, Brown.

98 **Racism plays a big role:** Terry, R. (2020, February 26). *How Black Culinary Historians Are Rewriting the History of American Food*. Yes! Solutions Journalism. https://www.yesmagazine.org/social-justice/2020/02/26/food-african-american-history.

98 **adults with disordered eating:** Alberts, H. J. E. M., Thewissen, R., and Raes, L. (2012). Dealing with problematic eating behaviour. The effects of a mindfulness-based intervention on eating behaviour, food cravings, dichotomous thinking and body image concern. *Appetite*, *58*(3), 847–851. https://doi.org/10.1016/J.APPET.2012.01.009; Antoniou, E. E., Bongers, P., and Jansen, A. (2017). The mediating role of dichotomous thinking and emotional eating in the relationship between depression and BMI. *Eating Behaviors*, *26*, 55–60. https://doi.org/10.1016/J.EATBEH.2017.01.007; Lakritz et al. (2022); Linardon, J., Messer, M., Helms, E. R., McLean, C., Incerti, L., and Fuller-Tyszkiewicz, M. (2020). Interactions between different eating patterns on recurrent binge-eating behavior: A machine learning approach. *International Journal of Eating Disorders*, *53*(4), 533–540. https://doi.org/10.1002/EAT.23232; Linardon, J., and Mitchell, S. (2017). Rigid dietary control, flexible dietary control, and intuitive eating: Evidence for their differential relationship to disordered eating and body image concerns. *Eating Behaviors*, *26*, 16–22. https://doi.org/10.1016/j.eatbeh.2017.01.008; Palascha, A., Van Kleef, E., and Van Trijp, H. C. M. (2015). How does thinking in Black and White terms relate to eating behavior and weight regain? *Journal of Health Psychology*, *20*(5), 638–648. https://doi.org/10.1177/1359105315573440.

98 **hypothesized that rather:** Eck, K. M., Quick, V., and Byrd-Bredbenner, C. (2022). Body dissatisfaction, eating styles, weight-related behaviors, and health among young women in the United States. *Nutrients*, *14*(18), 3876. https://doi.org/10.3390/NU14183876; Lakritz et al. (2022); Levinson, J. A., Parker, J. E., Hunger, J. M., and Tomiyama, A. J. (2025). Dichotomous thinking about food as an understudied subclinical disordered eating cognition. *Journal of Eating Disorders*, *13*(1). https://doi.org/10.1186/S40337-025-01388-7.

98 **research related to eating disorder prevention:** Berge, J. M., Hazzard, V. M., Arlinghaus, K. R., Larson, N., Hahn, S. L., and Neumark-Sztainer, D. (2024). Do parents engage in weight- and health-focused conversations with their emerging adult children and are there cross-sectional associations with weight and well-being outcomes? *Preventive Medicine*, *186*, 108066. https://doi.org/10.1016/j.ypmed.2024.108066; García-Muñoz, S., Barlińska, J., Wojtkowska, K., et al. (2022). Is it possible to improve healthy food habits in schoolchildren? A cross cultural study among Spain and Poland. *Food Quality and Preference*, *99*. https://doi.org/10.1016/j.foodqual.2022

.104534; Gold, A., Larson, M., Tucker, J., and Strang, M. (2017). Classroom nutrition education combined with fruit and vegetable taste testing improves children's dietary intake. *Journal of School Health*, *87*(2), 106–113. https://doi.org/10.1111/josh.12478; Gripshover, S. J., and Markman, E. M. (2013). Teaching young children a theory of nutrition. *Psychological Science*, *24*(8), 1541–1553. https://doi.org/10.1177/0956797612474827; Hasan, F., Nguyen, A. V., Reynolds, A. R., et al. (2023). Preschool- and childcare center–based interventions to increase fruit and vegetable intake in preschool children in the United States: A systematic review of effectiveness and behavior change techniques. *International Journal of Behavioral Nutrition and Physical Activity*, *20*(1), 1–12. https://doi.org/10.1186/S12966-023-01472-8/TABLES/1; Herzer, M., Zeller, M. H., Rausch, J. R., and Modi, A. C. (2011). Perceived social support and its association with obesity-specific health-related quality of life. *Journal of Developmental and Behavioral Pediatrics*, *32*(3), 188. https://doi.org/10.1097/DBP.0B013E318208F576; Holley, C. E., Haycraft, E., and Farrow, C. (2020). Unpacking the relationships between positive feeding practices and children's eating behaviours: The moderating role of child temperament. *Appetite*, *147*, 104548. https://doi.org/10.1016/j.appet.2019.104548; Jung, T., Huang, J., Eagan, L., and Oldenburg, D. (2019). Influence of school-based nutrition education program on healthy eating literacy and healthy food choice among primary school children. *International Journal of Health Promotion and Education*, *57*(2), 67–81. https://doi.org/10.1080/14635240.2018.1552177; Karpouzis, F., Anastasiou, K., Lindberg, R., Walsh, A., Shah, S., and Ball, K. (2025). Effectiveness of school-based nutrition education programs that include environmental sustainability components, on fruit and vegetable consumption of 5–12 year old children: A systematic review. *Journal of Nutrition Education and Behavior*. https://doi.org/10.1016/j.jneb.2025.02.008; Katz, D. L., Katz, C. S., Treu, J. A., et al. (2011). Teaching healthful food choices to elementary school students and their parents: The Nutrition Detectives™ program. *Journal of School Health*, *81*(1), 21–28. https://doi.org/10.1111/j.1746-1561.2010.00553.x; Koreshe, E., Paxton, S., Miskovic-Wheatley, J., et al. (2023). Prevention and early intervention in eating disorders: Findings from a rapid review. *Journal of Eating Disorders*, *11*(1). https://doi.org/10.1186/s40337-023-00758-3; Lwin, M. O., Shin, W., Yee, A. Z. H., and Wardoyo, R. J. (2017). A parental health education model of children's food consumption: Influence on children's attitudes, intention, and consumption of healthy and unhealthy foods. *Journal of Health Communication*, *22*(5), 403–412. https://doi.org/10.1080/10810730.2017.1302523; Medeiros, G. C. B. S. de, Azevedo, K. P. M. de, Garcia, D., et al. (2022). Effect of school-based food and nutrition education interventions on the food consumption of adolescents: A systematic review and meta-analysis. *International Journal of Environmental Research and Public Health*, *19*(17). https://doi.org/10.3390/IJERPH191710522; Melbye, E. L., and Hansen, H. (2015). Promotion and prevention focused feeding strategies: Exploring the effects on healthy and unhealthy child eating. *BioMed Research International*, 306306. https://doi.org/10.1155/2015/306306; Mora, M., Penelo, E., Gutiérrez, T., Espinoza, P., González, M. L., and Raich, R. M. (2015). Assessment of two school-based programs to prevent universal eating disorders: Media literacy and theatre-based methodology in Spanish adolescent boys and girls. *Scientific World Journal*. https://doi.org/10.1155/2015/328753; Muzaffar, H., Difilipo, K. N., Fitzgerald, N., et al. (2024). A systematic review of interventions to improve the diet of children. *Journal of Public Health (Germany)*. https://doi.org/10.1007/s10389-024-02258-3; Raich, R. M., Portell, M., and Peláez-Fernández, M. A. (2010). Evaluation of a school-based programme of universal eating disorders prevention: Is it more effective in girls at risk? *European Eating Disorders Review: The Journal of the Eating Disorders Association*, *18*(1), 49–57. https://doi.org/10.1002/ERV.968; Toh, J. Y., Quah, P. L., Wong, C. H., et al. (2021). Evaluation of a child food reward task and its association with maternal feeding practices. *PLOS One*, *16*(7). https://doi.org/10.1371/JOURNAL.PONE.0254773; Vaughan, K. L., Vidal, M., Cade, J. E., Hetherington, M. M., and Evans, C. E. L. (2025). Evaluation of the school-based "PhunkyFoods" intervention: A cluster randomised controlled trial in the UK. *Public Health Nutrition*, *28*(1), e86. https://doi.org/10.1017/S1368980025000552; Verdonschot, A., Follong, B. M., Collins, C. E., De Vet, E., Haveman-Nies, A., and Bucher, T. (2023). Effectiveness of school-based nutrition intervention components on fruit and vegetable intake and nutrition knowledge in children aged 4–12 years old: An umbrella review. *Nutrition Reviews*, *81*(3), 304. https://doi.org/10.1093/NUTRIT/NUAC057; Warschburger, P. and Zitzmann, J. (2018). The efficacy of a universal school-based prevention program for eating disorders among German adolescents: Results from a randomized-controlled trial. *Journal of Youth and Adolescence*, 47(6), 1317–1331. https://doi.org/10.1007/S10964-018-0852-3; Wong, R. S., Chan, B. N. K., Lai, S. I., and Tung, K. T. S. (2024). School-based eating disorder prevention programmes and their impact on adolescent mental health: Systematic review. *BJPsych Open*, *10*(6), e196. https://doi.org/10.1192/bjo.2024.795; Yee et al. (2017).

98 **If a child is very embodied:** Binder, A., Naderer, B., and Matthes, J. (2020b). The effects of gain- and loss-framed nutritional messages on children's healthy eating behaviour. *Public Health Nutrition*, *23*(10), 1726–1734. https://doi.org/10.1017/S1368980019004683; Bryan, C. J., Yeager, D. S., Hinojosa, C. P., et al. (2016). Harnessing adolescent values to motivate healthier eating. *Proceedings of the National Academy of Sciences of the United States of America*, *113*(39), 10830–10835. https://doi.org/10.1073/pnas.1604586113; DeJesus, J. M., Du, K. M., Shutts, K., and Kinzler, K. D. (2019). How information about what is "healthy" versus "unhealthy" impacts children's consumption of otherwise identical foods. *Journal of Experimental Psychology: General*, *148*(12), 2091–2103. https://doi.org/10.1037/xge0000588; Nicholson, J. S., Barton, J. M., and Simons, A. L. (2018).

Ability to categorize food predicts hypothetical food choices in Head Start preschoolers. *Journal of Nutrition Education and Behavior*, *50*(3), 238–246. e1. https://doi.org/10.1016/j.jneb.2017.09.026.
99 **This is not an official:** Brytek-Matera, A., and Donini, L. M. (2025). The need for research on orthorexia nervosa: looking back, looking forward. *Eating and Weight Disorders*, *30*(1), 48. https://doi.org/10.1007/S40519-025-01743-2; Eckley, T., Quirk, S. E., Pasco, J. A., Messer, M., and Williams, L. J. (2025). Prevalence of orthorexia nervosa: A systematic review and meta-analysis protocol. *BMJ Open*, *15*(5). https://doi.org/10.1136/BMJOPEN-2024-096802; Moccia, L., Anesini, M. B., Callovini, T., et al. (2025). Understanding orthorexia nervosa: A systematic review of meta-analytical findings. *Current Nutrition Reports*, *14*(1), 126. https://doi.org/10.1007/S13668-025-00714-4.
100 **seeing bright colors, logos, and smiling faces:** Kelly, B., Boyland, E., King, L., Bauman, A., Chapman, K., and Hughes, C. (2019). Children's exposure to television food advertising contributes to strong brand attachments. *International Journal of Environmental Research and Public Health*, *16*(13). https://doi.org/10.3390/ijerph16132358; Naderer, B., Binder, A., Matthes, J., and Mayrhofer, M. (2020). Healthy, sweet, brightly colored, and full of vitamins: Cognitive and affective persuasive cues of food placements and children's healthy eating behavior. *International Journal of Advertising*, *39*(7), 1012–1030. https://doi.org/10.1080/02650487.2020.1735140; Packer, J., Croker, H., Goddings, A. L., et al. (2022). Advertising and young people's critical reasoning abilities: Systematic review and meta-analysis. *Pediatrics*, *150*(6). https://doi.org/10.1542/peds.2022-057780.
100 **the tobacco industry:** Harris, J. L. (2020). Targeted food marketing to Black and Hispanic Consumers: The tobacco playbook. *American Journal of Public Health*, *110*(3), 271–272. https://doi.org/10.2105/AJPH.2019.305518.
101 **Many tobacco companies:** Fazzino, T. L., Jun, D., Chollet-Hinton, L., and Bjorlie, K. (2024). US tobacco companies selectively disseminated hyper-palatable foods into the US food system: Empirical evidence and current implications. *Addiction*, *19*(1), 62–71. https://doi.org/10.1111/add.16332; Harris (2020); Nguyen, K. H., Glantz, S. A., Palmer, C. N., and Schmidt, L. A. (2020). Transferring racial/ethnic marketing strategies from tobacco to food corporations: Philip Morris and Kraft General Foods. *American Journal of Public Health*, *110*(3), 329–336. https://doi.org/10.2105/AJPH.2019.305482.
101 **Advertising has also:** Boyland, E. J., Nolan, S., Kelly, B., et al. (2016). Advertising as a cue to consume: A systematic review and meta-analysis of the effects of acute exposure to unhealthy food and nonalcoholic beverage advertising on intake in children and adults. *American Journal of Clinical Nutrition*, *103*(2), 519–533. https://doi.org/10.3945/ajcn.115.120022; Bruce, A. S., Pruitt, S. W., Ha, O. R., et al. (2016). The influence of televised food commercials on children's food choices: Evidence from ventromedial prefrontal

cortex activations. *Journal of Pediatrics*, 177, 27–32.e1. https://doi.org/10.1016/j.jpeds.2016.06.067; Norman, J., Kelly, B., McMahon, A. T., et al. (2018). Children's self-regulation of eating provides no defense against television and online food marketing. *Appetite*, *125*, 438–444. https://doi.org/10.1016/j.appet.2018.02.026.

107 **adolescents to be able to:** Harris, J. L., Brownell, K. D., and Bargh, J. A. (2009). The food marketing defense model: Integrating psychological research to protect youth and inform public policy. *Social Issues and Policy Review*, *3*(1), 211–271. https://doi.org/10.1111/j.1751-2409.2009.01015.

107 **wouldn't expect kids under fourteen:** Packer, J., Croker, H., Goddings, A. L., et al. (2022). Advertising and young people's critical reasoning abilities: Systematic review and meta-analysis. *Pediatrics*, *150*(6). https://doi.org/10.1542/peds.2022-057780.

107 **Canada's national food guide:** Health Canada. (n.d.). Limit kids' exposure to food marketing. *Canada's Food Guide*. Retrieved February 3, 2024, from https://food-guide.canada.ca/en/healthy-eating-recommendations/marketing-can-influence-your-food-choices/limiting-kids-exposure-to-food-marketing/#section-3.

107 **potentially lessen the effects:** Binder, A., and Matthes, J. (2023). What can stop the "pester power"? A longitudinal study on the impact of children's audiovisual media consumption on media-motivated food purchase requests. *Pediatric Obesity*, *18*(6). https://doi.org/10.1111/ijpo.13018; Harris, J. L., Brownell, K. D., and Bargh, J. A. (2009). The food marketing defense model: Integrating psychological research to protect youth and inform public policy. *Social Issues and Policy Review*, *3*(1), 211–271. https://doi.org/10.1111/j.1751-2409.2009.01015.; Packer et al. (2022).

107 **you might use language:** Binder and Matthes (2023); Harris et al. (2009); Rozendaal, E., Buijs, L., and van Reijmersdal, E. A. (2016). Strengthening children's advertising defenses: The effects of forewarning of commercial and manipulative intent. *Frontiers in Psychology*, 7. https://doi.org/10.3389/fpsyg.2016.01186.

107 **Educating a child:** Binder and Matthes (2023); Harris et al. (2009).

108 **this marketing technique:** Harris et al. (2009).

108 **appealing to middle school-aged:** Bryan, C. J., Yeager, D. S., and Hinojosa, C. P. (2019). A values-alignment intervention protects adolescents from the effects of food marketing. *Nature Human Behaviour*, *3*(6), 596–603. https://doi.org/10.1038/s41562-019-0586-6.

110 **Share interesting facts:** Gripshover, S. J., and Markman, E. M. (2013). Teaching young children a theory of nutrition. *Psychological Science*, *24*(8), 1541–1553. https://doi.org/10.1177/0956797612474827.

110 **foods are morally neutral:** Yee et al. (2017).

110 **engaging experiences:** Inácio, M. L. C., Pereira, F. C., Fernandes, L. B., Oliveira, I. R. C. de, Pereira, R. C., and de Angelis-Pereira, M. C. (2022). Food and nutrition education using intuitive method and NOVA food classification: Implications for food practices of children and adolescents intuitive

method in food and nutrition education. *American Journal of Health Promotion*, *36*(7), 1170–1182. https://doi.org/10.1177/08901171221092394; Murimi, M. W., Moyeda-Carabaza, A. F., Nguyen, B., Saha, S., Amin, R., and Njike, V. (2018). Factors that contribute to effective nutrition education interventions in children: A systematic review. *Nutrition Reviews*, *76*(8), 553–580. https://doi.org/10.1093/nutrit/nuy020.

5: Eat What Nourishes Us

124 **Here's a general range:** Ajomiwe, N., Boland, M., Phongthai, S., Bagiyal, M., Singh, J., and Kaur, L. (2024). Protein nutrition: Understanding structure, digestibility, and bioavailability for optimal health. *Foods*, *13*(11). https://doi.org/10.3390/foods13111771; Hudson, J. L., Baum, J. I., Diaz, E. C., and Børsheim, E. (2021). Dietary protein requirements in children: Methods for consideration. *Nutrients*, *13*(5). https://doi.org/10.3390/nu13051554.

126 **serving them low-mercury fatty fish:** National Academies of Sciences. (2024). *The Role of Seafood Consumption in Child Growth and Development*. National Academies Press. https://doi.org/10.17226/27623.

126 **Fiber and your child's:** Basuray, N., Deehan, E. C., Vieira, F. T., et al. (2024). Dichotomous effect of dietary fiber in pediatrics: A narrative review of the health benefits and tolerance of fiber. *European Journal of Clinical Nutrition*, *78*(7), 557–568. https://doi.org/10.1038/S41430-024-01429-5; Kranz, S., Brauchla, M., Slavin, J. L., and Miller, K. B. (2012). What do we know about dietary fiber intake in children and health? The effects of fiber intake on constipation, obesity, and diabetes in children. *Advances in Nutrition*, *3*(1), 47–53). https://doi.org/10.3945/an.111.001362; Salvatore, S., Battigaglia, M. S., Murone, E., Dozio, E., Pensabene, L., and Agosti, M. (2023). Dietary fibers in healthy children and in pediatric gastrointestinal disorders: A practical guide. *Nutrients*, *15*(9), 2208. https://doi.org/10.3390/NU15092208; Veronese, N., Solmi, M., Caruso, M. G., et al. (2018). Dietary fiber and health outcomes: An umbrella review of systematic reviews and meta-analyses. *American Journal of Clinical Nutrition*, *107*(3), 436–444. https://doi.org/10.1093/ajcn/nqx082.

126 **Ninety-five percent:** 2025 Dietary Guidelines Advisory Committee. (2024). *Scientific Reports of the 2025 Dietary Guidelines Advisory Committee: Part D. Chapter 1: Current Dietary Intakes and Prevalence of Nutrition-Related Chronic Health Conditions*. U.S. Department of Health and Human Services.

127 **sugar-sweetened beverages are associated:** Onni, A. T., Balakrishna, R., Perillo, M., et al. (2025). Umbrella review of systematic reviews and meta-analyses on consumption of different food groups and risk of all-cause mortality. *Advances in Nutrition*, *16*(4). https://doi.org/10.1016/j.advnut.2025.100393

127 **as well as reducing:** Houlihan, J., and Brody, C. (2019). *What's in My Baby's Food?* Healthy Babies Bright Futures.

128 **the national regulation levels:** US Environmental Protection Agency.

(2025). *Consumer Confidence Reports.* https://www.epa.gov/ccr/ccr-information-consumers.

128 **One is high-mercury:** US Food and Drug Administration. (2024a, March). *Advice About Eating Fish.* US Food and Drug Administration. https://www.fda.gov/food/consumers/advice-about-eating-fish.

128 **Spices and imported candy:** US Food and Drug Administration. (2024b, December). *Lead in Food and Foodwares.* https://www.fda.gov/food/environmental-contaminants-food/lead-food-and-foodwares.

128 **They are classified:** International Agency for Research on Cancer. (2018). *Red Meat and Processed Meat: IARC Monographs on the Evaluation of Carcinogenic Risks to Humans*; Ungvari, Z., Fekete, M., Varga, P., et al. (2025). Association between red and processed meat consumption and colorectal cancer risk: A comprehensive meta-analysis of prospective studies. *GeroScience*, *47*(3), 5123. https://doi.org/10.1007/S11357-025-01646-1.

129 **The final foods:** Houlihan and Brody (2019).

130 **All kids need iron:** 2025 Dietary Guidelines Advisory Committee.

131 **due to the substantial:** Environmental Protection Agency. (2025). *Per- and Polyfluoroalkyl Substances (PFAS).* https://www.epa.gov/sdwa/and-polyfluoroalkyl-substances-pfas.

132 **over 60 percent of children:** 2025 Dietary Guidelines Advisory Committee.

132 **we want kids to eat 24 g:** Vos, M. B., Kaar, J. L., Welsh, J. A., et al. (2017). Added sugars and cardiovascular disease risk in children: A scientific statement from the American Heart Association. *Circulation*, *135*(19), e1017–e1034. https://doi.org/10.1161/CIR.0000000000000439/FORMAT/EPUB.

132 **Too many added sugars:** Bujtor, M., Turner, A. I., Torres, S. J., Esteban-Gonzalo, L., Pariante, C. M., and Borsini, A. (2021). Associations of dietary intake on biological markers of inflammation in children and adolescents: A systematic review. *Nutrients*, *13*(2), 1–29. https://doi.org/10.3390/NU13020356; Rupérez, A. I., Mesana, M. I., and Moreno, L. A. (2019). Dietary sugars, metabolic effects and child health. *Current Opinion in Clinical Nutrition and Metabolic Care*, *22*(3), 206–216. https://doi.org/10.1097/MCO.0000000000000553; Huang, Y., Chen, Z., Chen, B., et al. (2023). Dietary sugar consumption and health: Umbrella review. *BMJ (Clinical Research Ed.)*, *381*. https://doi.org/10.1136/BMJ-2022-071609.

132 **over 90 percent of kids:** 2025 Dietary Guidelines Advisory Committee.

132 **80 percent or more:** 2025 Dietary Guidelines Advisory Committee.

134 **the more plant foods:** McDonald, D., Hyde, E., Debelius, J. W., et al. (2018). American Gut: An open platform for citizen science microbiome research. *MSystems*, *3*(3), e00031-18. https://doi.org/10.1128/MSYSTEMS.00031-18.

141 **about 10 percent each day:** Miura, H., and Barlow, L. A. (2010). Taste bud regeneration and the search for taste progenitor cells. *Archives Italiennes de Biologie*, *148*(2), 107. https://pmc.ncbi.nlm.nih.gov/articles/PMC3545678/.

144 **During this pause:** Michael Caulfield, the developer of the SIFT method

of vetting information, calls this the "Stop" step (Stop, Investigate, Find, Trace); Van Kampen, K. (2023, September 7) Library guides: Evaluating resources and misinformation: The SIFT method. UChicago Library. https://guides.lib.uchicago.edu/c.php?g=1241077&p=9082322.

148 **we know from the data:** 2025 Dietary Guidelines Advisory Committee.

149 **the Food and Drug Administration:** National Center for Complementary and Integrative Health. (2019). *Using Dietary Supplements Wisely*. https://www.nccih.nih.gov/health/using-dietary-supplements-wisely.

7: Feeding Disagreements

169 **Being on the same page:** Gevers, D. W. M., van Assema, P., Sleddens, E. F. C., de Vries, N. K., and Kremers, S. P. J. (2015). Associations between general parenting, restrictive snacking rules, and adolescent's snack intake. The roles of fathers and mothers and interparental congruence. *Appetite*, *87*, 184–191. https://doi.org/10.1016/J.APPET.2014.12.220.

8: Starting the Eating Journey

189 **has changed consensus recommendations:** Fleischer, D. M., Chan, E. S., Venter, C., et al. (2021). A consensus approach to the primary prevention of food allergy through nutrition: Guidance from the American Academy of Allergy, Asthma, and Immunology; American College of Allergy, Asthma, and Immunology; and the Canadian Society for Allergy and Clinical Immunology; *The Journal of Allergy and Clinical Immunology in Practice*, *9*, 22-43.e4. https://doi.org/10.1016/j.jaip.2020.11.002.

192 **"as long as you can":** Gracner, T., Boone, C., and Gertler, P. J. (2024). Exposure to sugar rationing in the first 1000 days of life protected against chronic disease. *Science (New York)*, eadn5421. https://science.org/doi/10.1126/science.adn5421.

11: Extreme Picky Eating and ARFID

223 **the longer they have:** Cardona Cano, S., Tiemeier, H., Van Hoeken, D., et al. (2015). Trajectories of picky eating during childhood: A general population study. *International Journal of Eating Disorders*, *48*(6), 570–579. https://doi.org/10.1002/EAT.22384; Thompson, C., Cummins, S., Brown, T., and Kyle, R. (2015). What does it mean to be a "picky eater"? A qualitative study of food related identities and practices. *Appetite*, *84*, 235–239. https://doi.org/10.1016/J.APPET.2014.09.028.

224 **children with more "difficult temperaments":** Zohar, A. H., Pick, S., Lev-Ari, L., and Bachner-Melman, R. (2020). A longitudinal study of maternal feeding and children's picky eating. *Appetite*, *154*. https://doi.org/10.1016/j.appet.2020.104804.

225 **children experience these:** Chow, C. Y., Skouw, S., Bech, A. C., Olsen, A., and Bredie, W. L. P. (2022). A review on children's oral texture perception and preferences in foods. *Critical Reviews in Food Science and Nutrition*, *64*(12), 3861–3879. https://doi.org/10.1080/10408398.2022

.2136619; Jani, R., Irwin, C., Rigby, R., et al. (2024). Association between picky eating, weight status, vegetable, and fruit intake in children and adolescents: Systematic review and meta-analysis. *Childhood Obesity*. https://doi.org/10.1089/chi.2023.0196; van den Brand, A. J. P., Hendriks-Hartensveld, A. E. M., Havermans, R. C., et al. (2025). Food rejection is associated with tactile sensitivity and tactile appreciation in three-year-old children. *Appetite*, *204*, 107769. https://doi.org/10.1016/J.APPET.2024.107769.

225 **Kids with neurodivergence:** Adams, S. N. (2022). Feeding and swallowing issues in autism spectrum disorders. *Neuropsychiatric Disease and Treatment*, *18*, 2311. https://doi.org/10.2147/NDT.S332523; Harris, H. A., Bowling, A., Santos, S., Greaves-Lord, K., and Jansen, P. W. (2022). Child ADHD and autistic traits, eating behaviours and weight: A population-based study. *Pediatric Obesity*, 17(11), e12951. https://doi.org/10.1111/ijpo.12951; Zohar et al. (2020).

225 **These conditions can result:** Białek-Dratwa, A., Szymańska, D., Grajek, M., Krupa-Kotara, K., Szczepańska, E., and Kowalski, O. (2022). ARFID—Strategies for dietary management in children. *Nutrients*, *14*(9), 1739. https://doi.org/10.3390/NU14091739; Cardona Cano, S., Hoek, H. W., van Hoeken, D., et al. (2016). Behavioral outcomes of picky eating in childhood: A prospective study in the general population. *Journal of Child Psychology and Psychiatry, and Allied Disciplines*, *57*(11), 1239–1246. https://doi.org/10.1111/JCPP.12530; Chauhan, V. (2024). What's new in emergencies, trauma, and shock: Early recognition of scurvy in emergency departments can improve patient outcomes. *Journal of Emergencies, Trauma, and Shock*, 17(2), 51. https://doi.org/10.4103/JETS.JETS_71_24; del Campo, C., Bouzas, C., and Tur, J. A. (2024). Risk factors and consequences of food neophobia and pickiness in children and adolescents: A systematic review. *Foods (Basel, Switzerland)*, *14*(1), 69. https://doi.org/10.3390/FOODS14010069; James, R. M., O'Shea, J., Micali, N., Russell, S. J., and Hudson, L. D. (2024). Physical health complications in children and young people with avoidant restrictive food intake disorder (ARFID): A systematic review and meta-analysis. *BMJ Paediatrics Open*, *8*(1), e002595. https://doi.org/10.1136/bmjpo-2024-002595; Jani et al. (2024); Kells, M. R., Roske, C., Watters, A., et al. (2023). Vitamin D and hypophosphatemia in patients with anorexia nervosa and avoidant/restrictive food intake disorder: a case control study. *Journal of Eating Disorders*, *11*(1), 195. https://doi.org/10.1186/S40337-023-00913-W; Tanner, A. B., and Richmond, T. K. (2024). Assessing growth in children and adolescents with avoidant/restrictive food intake disorder. *Journal of Eating Disorders*, *12*(1), 82. https://doi.org/10.1186/s40337-024-01034-8; Taylor, C. M., Northstone, K., Wernimont, S. M., and Emmett, P. M. (2016). Macro- and micronutrient intakes in picky eaters: A cause for concern? *American Journal of Clinical Nutrition*, *104*(6), 1647. https://doi.org/10.3945/AJCN.116.137356; Taylor, C. M. and Emmett, P. M. (2019). Picky eating in children: Causes and consequences. *Pro-*

ceedings of the Nutrition Society, *78*(2), 161–169. https://doi.org/10.1017/S0029665118002586; Trapani, S., Rubino, C., Indolfi, G., and Lionetti, P. (2022). A narrative review on pediatric scurvy: The last twenty years. *Nutrients*, *14*(3), 684. https://doi.org/10.3390/NU14030684/S1.

225 **Their picky eating:** Taylor and Emmett (2019); Wolstenholme, H., Kelly, C., Hennessy, M., and Heary, C. (2020). Childhood fussy/picky eating behaviours: A systematic review and synthesis of qualitative studies. *International Journal of Behavioral Nutrition and Physical Activity*, *17*(1). https://doi.org/10.1186/s12966-019-0899-x.

226 **learned in family behavioral:** Białek-Dratwa et al. (2022); Peskin, A., Barth, A., Mansoor, E., et al. (2024). Impact of parent child interaction therapy on child eating behaviors. *Appetite*, *200*, 107544. https://doi.org/10.1016/j.appet.2024.107544; Reche-Olmedo, L., Torres-Collado, L., Compañ-Gabucio, L. M., and Garcia-De-la-hera, M. (2021). The role of occupational therapy in managing food selectivity of children with autism spectrum disorder: A scoping review. *Children*, *8*(11), 1024. https://doi.org/10.3390/children8111024.

12: When a Child Is Obsessed with Sweets, Can't Stop Eating Hyperpalatable Foods, or Is Sneaking Food

238 **reducing control over food:** Sonneville, K. R., Rifas-Shiman, S. L., Haines, J., et al. (2013). Associations of parental control of feeding with eating in the absence of hunger and food sneaking, hiding, and hoarding. *Childhood Obesity*, *9*(4), 346. https://doi.org/10.1089/CHI.2012.0149.

238 **including a lack of impulse control:** Reed, D. R., and McDaniel, A. H. (2006). The human sweet tooth. *BMC Oral Health*, *6* (Suppl 1), S17. https://doi.org/10.1186/1472-6831-6-S1-S17.

239 **Food preferences:** Alcock, J., Maley, C. C., and Aktipis, C. A. (2014). Is eating behavior manipulated by the gastrointestinal microbiota? Evolutionary pressures and potential mechanisms. *Bioessays*, *36*(10), 940. https://doi.org/10.1002/BIES.201400071.

239 **antibiotics may upset:** The relationship of gut microbiota and food preferences is an emerging area of research and, as such, it is still relies heavily on animal studies. Novelle, M. G. (2021). "Decoding the Role of Gut-Microbiome in the Food Addiction Paradigm." *International Journal of Environmental Research and Public Health*, *18*(13), 6825. https://doi.org/10.3390/IJERPH18136825; Ousey, J., Boktor, J. C., and Mazmanian, S. K. (2023). Gut microbiota suppress feeding induced by palatable foods. *Current Biology*, *33*(1), 147-157.e7. https://doi.org/10.1016/J.CUB.2022.10.066; Zhang, T., Wang, W., Li, J., et al. (2025). Free fatty acid receptor 4 modulates dietary sugar preference via the gut microbiota. *Nature Microbiology*, *10*(2), 348–361. https://doi.org/10.1038/S41564-024-01902-8.

14: Health Diagnoses and Therapeutic Diets

275 **dyes can have visible:** de Oliveira, Z. B., Silva da Costa, D. V., da Silva

dos Santos, A. C., et al. (2024). Synthetic colors in food: A warning for children's health. *International Journal of Environmental Research and Public Health, 21*(6), 682. https://doi.org/10.3390/IJERPH21060682.

287 **Many eating disorder therapists:** National Alliance for Eating Disorders. (2023). *To the Members of the American Academy of Pediatrics.* https://www.allianceforeatingdisorders.com/american-academy-pediatrics/.

287 **some research to suggest:** Jebeile, H., Gow, M. L., Baur, L. A., Garnett, S. P., Paxton, S. J., and Lister, N. B. (2019). Treatment of obesity, with a dietary component, and eating disorder risk in children and adolescents: A systematic review with meta-analysis. *Obesity Reviews, 20*(9), 1287. https://doi.org/10.1111/OBR.12866.

289 **newer clinical trial data:** Fox, C. K., Barrientos-Pérez, M., Bomberg, E. M., et al. (2024). Liraglutide for children 6 to ‹12 years of age with obesity—A randomized trial. *New England Journal of Medicine.* https://doi.org/10.1056/NEJMOA2407379.

289 **small amount of research:** Fox et al. (2024). Katole, N. T., Salankar, H. V., et al. (2024). The antiobesity effect and safety of GLP-1 receptor agonist in overweight/obese adolescents without diabetes mellitus: A systematic review and meta-analysis. *Cureus, 16*(8), e66280. https://doi.org/10.7759/CUREUS.66280; Liu, L., Shi, H., Shi, Y., et al. (2024). Comparative efficacy and safety of glucagon-like peptide-1 receptor agonists in children and adolescents with obesity or overweight: A systematic review and network meta-analysis. *Pharmaceuticals (Basel, Switzerland), 17*(7). https://doi.org/10.3390/PH17070828.

290 **Researchers have observed:** Koreshe, E., Paxton, S., Miskovic-Wheatley, J., et al. (2023). Prevention and early intervention in eating disorders: Findings from a rapid review. *Journal of Eating Disorders, 11*(1). https://doi.org/10.1186/s40337-023-00758-3.

Appendix

303 **Fiber recommendations:** Institute of Medicine (2005). *Dietary reference intakes for energy, carbohydrate, fiber, fat, fatty acids, cholesterol, protein, and amino acids.* National Academies Press. https://doi.org/10.17226/10490; Kranz, S., Brauchla, M., Slavin, J. L., and Miller, K. B. (2012). What do we know about dietary fiber intake in children and health? The effects of fiber intake on constipation, obesity, and diabetes in children. *Advances in Nutrition, 3*(1), 47–53. https://doi.org/10.3945/an.111.001362; Salvatore, S., Battigaglia, M. S., Murone, E., Dozio, E., Pensabene, L., and Agosti, M. (2023). Dietary fibers in healthy children and in pediatric gastrointestinal disorders: A practical guide. *Nutrients, 15*(9), 2208. https://doi.org/10.3390/nu15092208; Williams, C. L., Bollella, M., and Wynder, E. L. (1995). A new recommendation for dietary fiber in childhood. *Pediatrics, 96*(5 Pt 2), 985–988.

304 **Calcium recommendations:** Cormick, G., and Belizán, J. M. (2019). Calcium intake and health. *Nutrients, 11*(7), 1606. https://doi.org/10.3390

/nu11071606; Institute of Medicine. (2011). *Dietary reference intakes for calcium and vitamin D.* National Academies Press. https://doi.org/10.17226/13050; EFSA Panel on Dietetic Products, Nutrition and Allergies. (2015). Scientific opinion on dietary reference values for calcium. *EFSA Journal, 13*(5), 4101. https://doi.org/10.2903/j.efsa.2015.4101; World Health Organization & Food and Agriculture Organization of the United Nations. (2004). *Vitamin and mineral requirements in human nutrition (2nd ed.).* WHO. https://www.who.int/publications/i/item/9241546123.

306 **Iron recommendations:** Institute of Medicine. (2001). *Dietary reference intakes for vitamin A, vitamin K, arsenic, boron, chromium, copper, iodine, iron, manganese, molybdenum, nickel, silicon, vanadium, and zinc.* National Academies Press. https://doi.org/10.17226/10026.

INDEX

ABOUT THE AUTHOR

Jennifer Anderson, MSPH, RDN, is the founder of Kids Eat in Color, a trusted comprehensive resource for parents supporting their child's nutrition and relationship with food, with a social media audience of more than two million. She is the CEO of BetterBites®, a platform of digital health programs that equip parents with tools to guide their children through nutrition-related diagnoses and challenges. She is a registered dietitian and has a master of science in public health from the Johns Hopkins Bloomberg School of Public Health. She lives in Maryland with her husband and two kids.